SEMANTIC AND PRAGMATIC LANGUAGE DISORDERS

Assessment and Remediation

Ellyn V. Lucas, Ed.D.

Assistant Professor
Speech Pathology/Audiology Department
Texas Tech University
Lubbock, Texas

AN ASPEN PUBLICATION®
Aspen Systems Corporation
Rockville, Maryland
London
1980

Library of Congress Cataloging in Publication Data

Lucas, Ellyn V.
Semantic and pragmatic language disorders.

Includes bibliographies and index.
1. Language disorders in children. 2. Semantics.
3. Pragmatics. I. Title.
RJ496.L35L82   618.92'855   80-24120
ISBN: 0-89443-327-X

Library of Congress Catalog Card Number: 80-24120
ISBN: 0-89443-327-X

Printed in the United States of America

1 2 3 4 5

To my family

Table of Contents

Preface

This book is written for people who work with language disordered children. The material has been developed for the language clinicians, educators, and parents who need to have someone else synthesize the literature and from it make practical suggestions about remediation techniques and procedures.

The book is intended to meet several needs often expressed by individuals who work with language disordered children. These needs have been verbalized by workshop participants and college students and have been corroborated by my observations in schools and clinics. The following list summarizes these needs:

- There's too much literature on language development and theory, and I don't have enough background to apply the material.

- My children's language does not follow the normal developmental charts of language acquisition.

- The current assessment procedures don't tell me what is wrong with the child's language.

- My children's language is not delayed; it's weird.''

- I can't use these sophisticated programs that take the child through syntax and morphology up to embedding and conjoining; I would be pleased if my children could just use language to meet basic needs.

- I have children who respond beautifully to the language program tasks but never really get better at communicating.

- I have a child who doesn't make sense when he talks. He's passing all of the language tests at his age level, but there is something wrong with his language.

- The material on pragmatics and semantics is really interesting but I'm confused about application.

- When do I teach syntax, or should all of my children be on a semantic program?

- I can't handle a group of language disordered children because their attention spans are too short.

The list of complaints continues, but these are the concerns voiced most frequently. From my work as a clinician, consultant of language, university professor, and clinical supervisor, these complaints are warranted.

In this book I have attempted to solve some of these complaints by providing direct application procedures for specific language behaviors believed to be representative of language disorders. I have limited the theory and literature review and have emphasized the application of basic principles. I have offered alternative methods for assessing language disordered children and have explained the processes for accountability. Finally, I have couched these practical suggestions in a theoretical framework that suggests that communication is the ultimate goal of any language therapy for language disordered children.

By attempting to synthesize my knowledge into workable ideas for others, there are three basic professional risks: (1) There may be a tendency to overestimate the importance of one perspective in lieu of other ideas; (2) There may be too much synthesizing so that the theoretical premise is weakened; and (3) The desire to integrate ideas may lead the reader to underestimate the significance of specific theoretical principles and issues. I recognize these risks and respond to them by requesting that colleagues do research to support, reject, or alter any of the material presented here. Only through a willingness to share and research ideas can the quality of knowledge be improved.

At this time, my paramount goal is to meet the needs of the practitioner, the person who has to work with language disordered children. I know that my ideas have been effective for many clients, students, clinicians, educators, and parents. And I know it's time to deal with language disorders from a practical and logical perspective. If this book is of benefit to some of the individuals who work with language disordered children—if this book leads to improved remediation—then my purpose will have been accomplished.

Ellyn V. Lucas
Lubbock, Texas
October 1980

Acknowledgments

I wish to thank the friends and family who contributed their time and support to this endeavor. Without their insistence, I would not have made the time to do it. I also wish to thank Joyce Metz Roberts for handling the manuscript and Dr. Cran Lucas for his professional support.

CHAPTER OBJECTIVES

- explain the theorized development of specific types of referents, including those related to adult nouns, verbs, and dimensional terms.

- discuss the relationship between referential meaning and vocabulary acquisition.

- explain referential meaning and its process of acquisition.

- outline the theoretical issues of comprehension, imitation, and production as each pertains to semantic language acquisition.

- define the terms *predication, proposition, modulation,* and *referring,* and discuss each term's significance in the language acquisition process of young children.

- explain the basic semantic relations most frequently used in children's language.

- give examples of prelinguistic intention-based behavior.

- list and define the conventional set of symbols used for linguistic communication.

- explain the difference between direct and elicited or spontaneous imitation.

- explain the significant variables of a child's environment for language acquisition.

- explain the relationship between intended behavior and language development.

Chapter 1

Semantic Development and Its Importance to Language Intervention

The wonder and complexity of language must not be allowed to mask the simplicity of its purpose!

AN OVERVIEW OF SEMANTIC DEVELOPMENT

The purpose of providing an overview of semantic development is to suggest a theoretical basis for the assessment procedures and intervention strategies discussed in later chapters. This chapter does not present an exhaustive listing of the literature regarding semantics since many good reviews of psycholinguistic and sociolinguistic research are available (e.g., Clark & Clark, 1977; Foss & Hakes, 1978; Leonard, 1976; Moerk, 1977; Moore, 1973; Ochs & Schieffelin, 1979). However, an overview of the relevant points of normal semantic development is supportive of the basic tenet of this book: that the remediation process for language disorders should be approached from what is known about normal development, with the knowledge from normal development being blended with what is known about each exceptional child's special needs.

The material in this chapter is based on the premise that a child's semantic acquisition parallels observed patterns of behavior that reflect a child's level of cognitive development. Thus the child's cognitive and semantic development provides the basis for the linguistic patterns expressed by the conventional, phonological, and morphological rules used to formulate syntactical constructions.

Experience Basis

Each child brings an inmate, genetic endowment to an environment that is unique and perpetually changing. At birth the infant is quickly incorporated

1

into the environment as a manipulator as well as a receiver of others' actions and objects. As the child becomes actively incorporated into a unique and individualized environment, an assimilation of the endless changes ensues. Consequently the child shares through association bonds, these experiences with the significant people.

The sharing of experiences, by necessity, provides an overlap of common people, objects, and actions that are considered to be joint experiences between the child and the significant others (Bruner, 1974). During personal experience, the objects, actions, and events are linguistically specified by the adults. For example, "Let's take a bath" specifies the action and event for the child in conventional *markers* or *lexicon* (vocabulary). The event of bathing becomes associated with the linguistic markers used by the adult so that the experience becomes a joint reference with the child. As shown in Figure 1-1, both individuals share the experience, referred to by a lexical item, *bath*, which is then associated to the event.

Referential Meaning

Through the joint interaction, the child learns the specific *referents* or *lexical tags* of objects, actions, and events as specified by adults. The form of the

Figure 1-1 Joint Reference between Child and Caretaker

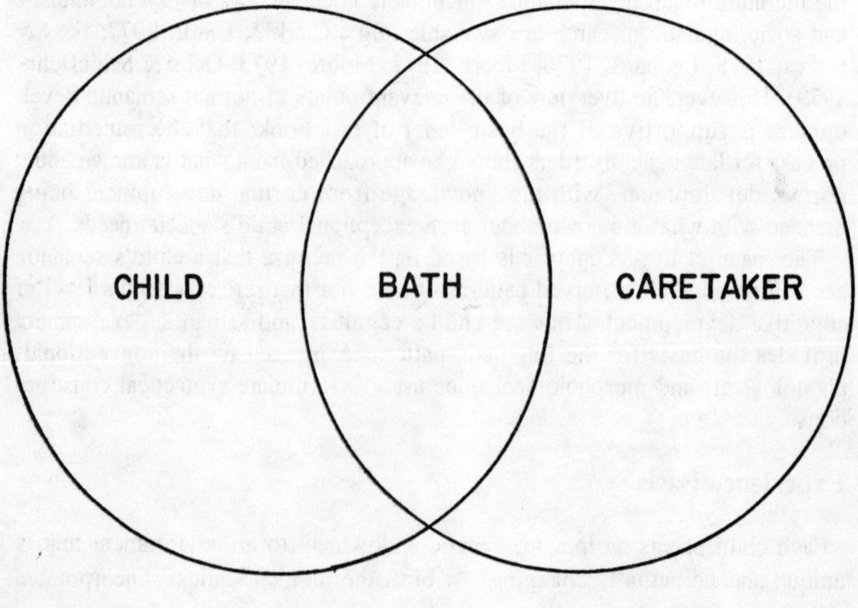

referent is presented in the conventional symbols including the sound system *(phonology)*, the elemental meaningful unit system *(morphology)*, and the order by which the units are joined *(syntax)*. The content of the symbols *(referential meaning)*, although expressed by a rule system, is established from the jointly shared experiences. The rules that govern linguistic behavior appear to be part of the child's innate ability to acquire language and are not a reduction of an adult formulation (Berko, 1958; Bloom, 1970; Brown, 1968). Through these interactions the child develops a system of symbols unique to his/her society.

The adults in discourse (Ervin-Tripp, 1978) with the child make constant use of the conventional symbols so that "marking the referents" or "referential meaning" is established. A referent exists only if the child and the adult, in either the hearer or speaker roles, have similar perceptual and functional experiences (E. Clark, 1974). The environments of the individual and the society merge as the culture is transmitted (Bernstein, 1967) through language.

Perceptual and functional knowledge is acquired through the interaction of the child in the environment, which has an impact on the cognitive physiological structures. This interaction between the environment and the child takes the form of sensory input (taste, touch, vision, audition, smell) that is processed through a series of sorting skills (discrimination) and integrating skills (perception). The integration of this perceptual material results in bits of semantic information or *semantic features* being cognitively recorded for future use.

When environmental information is meaningful to the child and is consistently processed in the same or similar units, this results in uniform behavior. For example, the infant begins sucking at the sight of the nipple because the perceptual characteristics of the object, the caretaker's actions, or the events are associated to functional characteristics that have been processed on previous occasions. Different nipples on different bottles are easily recognized as similar and thus produce consistent sucking behavior. But the same infant may be confused by the similarity between mama's voice and the voice of mama's sister. The infant's ability to differentiate between any male and female voice, or between two perceptually similar nipples, but not between two similar female voices is a temporary level of knowledge that consists of acquired semantic features. Experiences provide semantic bits of information for integration and processing, and this continuous building of information supplies the basis of lexical development.

Therefore, each lexical item is really a concept consisting of information from a variety of shared experiences between the child and significant others. These concepts constitute the referents to which a child or adult may refer. *Referring* is critical to the development of language since the ideas or thoughts that a child wishes to communicate must be expressable in common terms shared by the speaker and hearer. Hence, an object with similar perceptual and functional attributes must have a common label, such as "table." The common label or linguistic tag makes it possible for a speaker to refer to the object (table) with reasonable confidence that the hearer will have developed a joint referent from similar exposures.

Semantic Relations

The development of a repertoire of meaningful referents is crucial to a child's language development. This semantic acquisition of referents represents the organization between the child and the environment that is simplistically and relationally arranged and linguistically represented in the child's first one-term relations (Brown, 1973). These one-word or (more accurately) one-term semantic relations express a child's own perception (Schlesinger, 1974) of environmental conditions in relationship to people, objects, actions, and/or events. For example, a child says "milk" with a rising inflection and holds out a hand to receive the cup of milk that is sitting on the table. In this context the child's expression of the lexical item "milk" represents knowledge of semantic features both perceptual and functional. In this case, the child recognizes that the cup has milk (perceptual) and that drinking the milk would probably be enjoyable (functional). With the single lexical item, a relationship between the milk and the child is implied by the context; that is, the child expresses a present or immediate referent with appropriate *paralinguistic* aspects such as *prosody* or vocal patterns, gestures, and facial and body movements.

The hearer's understanding of the utterance "milk" is dependent on many other contextual variables that are not purely linguistic. The child's gestures and facial expressions are part of the total cultural form of communication. Learning to mark a referent must also be coupled with paralinguistic or nonlinguistic aspects for communication.

When two lexical items begin to be paired together (e.g., "milk," "drink"), then the child is coming closer to expressing direct linguistic relationships representative of the child's increasing underlying knowledge of the environment. There is a period of pausing that occurs between the one-term semantic relations and the two-term relations. The pause appears to represent a child's attempt to comment on the first term, but this is an adult's interpretation. The comma between the two terms ("milk," "drink") is used to indicate the proximity of the terms but does not necessarily express a direct relationship. Even when two terms are directly paired by context ("drink milk"), these pairings can be interpreted only for content and not for structure. Bloom (1970) shared a classic example of one utterance ("mommy sock") which, when produced in two different contexts, expressed two different semantic relationships. In one context, the utterance obviously referred to the idea of mommy putting on mommy's sock. In the other situation, mommy was obviously putting the child's sock on the child. These different meanings represented different underlying bits of knowledge but were expressed by the same linguistic construction. These types of semantic relations that represent underlying semantic (Schlesinger, 1974), cognitive (Nelson, 1973; Olson, 1970), knowledge may be differentiated on the basis of the child's intent. For example (Bloom, 1970), if mommy is putting on mommy's sock, then "mommy" is the actor or agent of the action to the object. The relationship might be expressed as "agent + object," but mommy could also show possession as "mommy's sock" or "possessive + X." If the utterance ("mommy sock") indicates that the child is receiving the action, then the semantic relationship is probably the same with underlying differences in knowledge. Without the context this underlying information would be underestimated, and the form of the utterance would be overgeneralized to equate adultlike utterances.

The adult who insists on ascribing adultlike construction labels to these early semantic relations runs the risk of selecting the wrong interpretation. For example, a clinician insisted that a particular child had syntactical problems because the child said "throw me" when the child wanted the ball. The clinician did not realize that there are at least two possibilities: "(You) throw (to) me the ball" and "I want you to throw (to me) the ball." In the latter case "me" would be in the wrong position, but in the first interpretation, the child's utterance ("throw me") was appropriate. Even when the context is known, the adult description of children's utterances must be considered from the semantic relations that the child demonstrates and not from pseudoadult rules that attempt to confine the child's language expression to adult structures.

The literature has described many of the semantic relations that children express. The most common relations (Bowerman, 1973; Brown, 1973; Leonard, 1976; Schlesinger, 1974) include the following intended information:

- "Agent + action" expresses the relationship between a person (agent) who is doing something and what that person is doing (action).

- "Action + object" expresses the relationship between the doing (action) and the recipient of the action (the object). There are also inanimate instruments that can function much like an agent.

- "Introducer + X" expresses the relationship between a lexical item that indicates any agent or object (X).

- "X + dative" or "dative + X" shows the relationship between the indirect recipient of an action and the object or agent. For example, "throw me" (meaning "throw me the ball") expresses the relationship between the indirect recipient "me" (the direct recipient is the understood "ball") and the action "throw." (Although the term *active* is a grammatical category, the variety of functions will be discussed in Chapter 2.)

- "X + locative" illustrates the relationship between any place (location) and an object or action or agent. For example, "Up mama" (to express that the child is being moved in an "up" direction) expresses the assumed relationship between the agent and the location of action (up). "Put ball" (to indicate that mama is putting the ball on the table) expresses the relationship between the action and the location of the object.

- "Modifier + X" expresses the relationship between a perceptual quality and an object, action, or agent. For example, "big ball" is the relationship between the object and some understanding of a size dimension. "Big kiss" may be attached to the action of kissing. "Big mommy" may be used by a child to indicate that one person is bigger than another. (The term *modifier* is also a grammatical term with a variety of purposes underlying its use.)

Although the two-term semantic relations listed above are the most common, a child might use other, nonstandard semantic relationships while developing the initial semantic basis. McLean and Snyder-McLean (1978) provide a checklist and methodology for assessing those semantic relations which the authors believe to be most important in a child's early language development. Since semantic relations are not regulated by *morphophonemic* or adultlike grammatical rules, it is prudent, for clinical purposes, to consider these earliest utterances in context and according to an assumed intended expression of specific knowledge about the environment.

From the child's expression of semantic relations the adult obtains insight into how the child interprets information in context. If the child uses a variety of the semantic relations, then the positive interaction between the child and adult supports and continues the language acquisition process. If the child does not use the expected semantic relations, the process is challenged and the substitutions are indicative of the child's learning difficulties. The use of those semantic relations denoting agents, actions, and objects are important and expressed most frequently by nonlanguage-delayed children, probably because the environment often functions in these relationships.

If a child does not use a variety of semantic relations (with particular emphasis on the frequency of types), then the child may be expressing psychosocial problems or a language disorder. Some children with poor self-awareness delete or avoid expressing relationships that use an agent. These children do not answer direct questions which imply that the child, an agent, will answer. The child who is in the "agent + X" relationship feels pressured, and the stress of the situation prevents the child from responding.

When "introducers + X" relationships (such as "This dog" or "This a dog" or "Here baby") dominate a child's language, then the functional appropriateness of that child's language must be considered and the environment that supports the language development must be examined carefully. The predominance of these relationships (at the expense of other relationships that reflect a child's interaction and manipulation of agents and objects) suggests an inadequate building of information or an inadequate semantic basis for later acquired linguistic skills. Examination of the child's environment frequently reveals that the child is receiving too much exposure for adultlike constructions (simple sentences) void of the underlying semantic basis critical to the child's acquisition of a semantic rule system for useful language development. The use of the introducer forms appears to be primarily at the expense of referent variety.

These early semantic relations consist almost entirely of referents that are *contentives* or content bearing words (Brown, 1973). To the child the words represent ideas or thoughts. The one or two words are individual units only to the adult; the child visualizes and acts upon a paragraph, a page, a book of words as one idea represented by a single-term relationship. As the child begins to initiate comments about referents, the lexical items of specification or function begin to emerge. These specification items, called *functors* (Brown, 1973), include articles such as "a" or "the," auxiliary verbs such as "is," and prepositions such as "in" or "on."

The functors cannot be visualized or represented by imagery in the same way as a referent or contentive can be represented. For example, "Show me *is*" is an impossible task. Functors assist in marking the contentives so that the child has the flexibility of the language. In the utterance "The lamps are big" the child specifies the referent "lamp" and illustrates the existing relationship between the size and the referent. The flexibility of the language explains the increase in saying more about thoughts or ideas already cognitively present. The child's novel utterances may be referred to as linguistic flexibility.

Predication and Modulation

When the child comments about a lamp in the example, "The lamp is big," a *predication* of the referent lamp is uttered. Predication, in simple terms, is the child's extension of a basic idea. For example, *lamp* is an idea that exists because a joint referent is established between the child and others. "The lamp is big" or "Big lamp" is therefore a predication of the referential meaning of lamp. The proposition or idea is grammatically expanded by the insertion of the functor *is* to "The lamp is big." The content of referring and/or predicating is known as the idea of the speaker or the proposition of the utterance.

The early development of semantic relations between the child and others provide a basis for modulating or changing the referential and/or meaning for specifying or making predications about the basic ideas. The forms of the adult societal speakers are acquired through the process of referring, predicating, and modulating. The *modulations* are changes in the language form made by introducing *morphemes* (basic units of meaning) that alter the substantive meaning. The intent of the utterance and the communicative purpose may be the same, but surface changes alter the meaning such that "dog" can be changed to plural "dogs" by adding the inflection morpheme *-s*. For an in-depth explanation of "modulation of meaning," see Brown (1973). Through the process of modulation the basic referents are changed to provide the adultlike flexibility of the language.

Flexibility of linguistic structures indicates that the speaker is able to say an infinite number of individualized and specific ideas in an infinite number of ways to match the variety of experiences that underlie the acquisition of knowledge. If the child's flexibility is reduced, the child's ability to express personal ideas is also diminished. The adult working with this child must decide: *Does the child's lack of flexibility represent a problem with learning or with producing the linguistic structures, or is the reduction of flexibility a product of a reduction in the information and understanding of perceptual and functional semantic knowledge?* Reduced expression, for whatever reason, may have more significant implications. The child's ability to produce ideas or thoughts may also be negatively affected since some theorists suggest that language facilitates thought (Vygotsky, 1934/1962) and that expression facilitates more language. From a clinical perspective, those children who are put into programs that emphasize expression do show quick gains in the linguistic flexibility and in the more advanced expression of their own intentions (Lucas, 1977).

The child's early semantic basis is modulated and subsequently expanded into more adultlike structures. This explanation is not meant to undermine the complex process but to describe what is occurring on the surface. For example, "Mommy go" (context provides agent + action experience) is changed to structures such as "Mommy going," "Mommy is going," "My mommy is going," and includes complex ideas such as "My mom is going to town to buy some clothes for my brother and me." The more complex structures are not simply mapped onto underlying semantic bases (Bowerman cited in Schlesinger, 1974; McLean & Snyder-McLean, 1978); the semantic information is increased as the structures are increased so that the form representing this information also increases in complexity. For example, Bloom, Miller, and Hood (1978) have discussed the semantic basis to the modulation of the verb. For example, "go" may be changed to "going" to represent the locative action meaning attached to the inflectional morpheme *-ing.* If the child does not have some of the semantic features (for example, location) of the verb concept, represented in the present progressive form by the morpheme *-ing,* the probability of using this morpheme is reduced. In other words, if a child has learned that "I ain't got no more pencils" means "I don't have any pencils," then the child will continue to use the learned or familiar structure because the meaning was originally attached to the familiar lexical items or the referential meaning. The child may understand the utterance "I don't have any pencils" just as the teacher understands "I ain't got no more pencils," but the latter usage constitutes the child's conventional set of meaningful symbols. Subsequently, changing the form to match the teacher's usage requires switching the child's code associated to the restricted context. It does not mean that the child's referential meaning is changed. A code switch denotes a variation in the representation and not necessarily an alternation of meaning. All speakers use variations in expression that are situation specific. Examples of common variations include "formalized" structure for authority figures such as the boss or the professor and "informal" structure and slang for peers and some family members.

The child's consistent and appropriate use of the morphemes that have been acquired through their meaning is significant to clinical application. For example, a child won't spontaneously use a present progressive verb (verbing) construction if the structure doesn't have meaning, even if the child can consistently respond with the grammatically desired form for a given task. The following lexical classes are marked by specific morphemes, which by definition of a morpheme do have meaning in their acquisition. Plurals are denoted by attaching a morpheme to indicate number. Prepositions represent the child's development of space and time. Pronouns denote person, gender, and number. Articles indicate general or specific objects. Auxiliary verbs and inflectional morphemes for verbs denote time and number. Even the form of the utterance signals the intent and restricts the purpose of the utterance, since the speaker produces either an interrogative, imperative, or declarative form.

SEMANTIC COGNITIVE DEVELOPMENT

The development of the referents in the language appears to parallel the level of cognitive processing or thinking as suggested by the epistemologist, Piaget (1971; Gruber & Voneche, 1977; and followers such as Sinclair-deZwart, 1973). The question of how this parallel process occurs—that is, whether cognition structures language or whether language structures cognition (Vygotsky, 1934/1962)—will not be answered here. From a clinical perspective, it appears that both processes may be occurring (Lewis & Brooks-Gunn, 1979). The following section describes the theoretical development of referents in language acquisition and is based on observation, research, and the literature.

Objective and Agentive Referents

The first type of referent to be discussed is the object, event, or person used by the infant to express the semantic relationship of the child to an agent or object. The class of words as interpreted by the adult grammarian is usually confined to the nouns. The development of these referents parallels the four basic stages of cognitive thinking (Piaget, 1971) and represents the underlying cognitive structures and their processes.

A common object, "bike" has been chosen to illustrate the hypothetical word development as outlined in Table 1-1. As the referential meaning of "bike" is traced through its development, the acquisition and specification of perceptual and functional features are apparent. Once a sufficient number of features have been acquired, the child is able to categorize the word "bike" into the category of transportation. This gradual process illustrates the importance of exposing a child to experiences in which the child may use the word in context. The feedback one gets from using the word in various settings helps the child sort out the valuable from the useless or conflicting information. Feedback or assistance is usually provided by an adult or caretaker who uses conventional symbols to linguistically mark the referents for the child. For example, the child points to the bird and says "uh." The parent says, "Yeah, that's Birdie—he is your bird. Grandpa gave Birdie to you. Say 'Hi,' Birdie, hi." The parent's natural reduction of structural complexity provides the child with simple input about the referent "bird." The parent also specified the referent "your birdie" and used the original referent "bird" to capitalize on a child's diminutive for a name, "Birdie."

The process of identifying the referent for the child and then attaching the appropriate linguistic term apparently marks the beginning of linguistic interaction between the caretaker and the child, or what may be referred to as *deixis* (Bruner, 1974-75). Deixis, or the communicative interaction between the infant and caretaker, incorporates language into the information-building process. Chapter 2 describes the social significance of deixis in the process of language acquisition.

As the deixis continues, the caretaker and child share multiple experiences that are constantly marked. The linguistic tags are subsequently learned through this natural social process. If the deixis ceases for any reason or if the amount of deixis is reduced, the impact (although immeasurable at this time) is going to be observable (Als, 1979; Wulbert, Inglis, Kriegsmann, & Mills, 1978). Reasons for interruption of the deixis include parent-to-child personality conflicts, an abnormal development in the child that reduces parent expectations and subsequent linguistic marking, and emotional or physical determinants. Since deixis is social in nature, the parent also expects something from the child. If the child is not progressing as expected (if the child doesn't respond when the parent talks), then the deixis is interrupted. Without the child to parent interaction, the number of referents and possibly the quality of referents for the noun class are reduced. Bretherton and Bates (1979, p. 96) have suggested that "vocabulary size and other strictly linguistic measures" are related to mother-child interaction.

Table 1-1 Development of a Referent of Agentive Objective Means

Approximate Age	Adult Question	Child's Response
0-2 Stage 1: Sensory to motor learning	"What's a bike?" "Where's your bike?" "Show me your bike?" "Do you have a bike?"	Same response; if a child has had a bike experience, then the child gets the bike or points to it or rides it, etc. The child's response is related to actual experience, and the adult expects a verbal or nonverbal label.
2-5 Stage 2: Perceptual and functional attributes are organized through experiences	Different questions receive different responses. "What is a bike?"	"Well, you ride it. My brother has a blue bike."
5-7	(Given a picture)	"This bike is like my bike."
7-11 Stage 3: Concepts are organized and related to experience	"What's a bike?"	"Well, it's got two wheels, you pedal it, it is used to get places, etc."
11+ Stage 4: Definitions consist of concept complexes	"What is a bike?"	"It's a cheap and healthy form of transportation."

Action Referents

For adults, the referents that describe action usually belong to the grammatical class of verbs, but for a child, action words don't have to be verbs. When semantic relations are expressed, the child might say "wagon" and intend for the adult to push. The adult will understand this request for action and push the child in the wagon. This interactive process assists the development of main verbs as referents, just as the process developed nouns as referents.

Actions are an integral part of a child's language learning. Early instinctive forms of reflex behavior, present at birth, give way to intended forms of action (Bates, Camaioni, & Volterra, 1975; Bruner, 1974-75) representative of the child's innate and learned abilities. Bruner (1973) analyzed children's intentions according to the features characterizing the act. These characteristics of action progress through several patterns. First, the child may gaze at an object or person and respond to it or to the event by excited and exaggerated motor behavior that cannot possibly allow the child to reach or grasp the object. Secondly, the child continues to try to achieve or obtain the object or act by motor skills that are being refined. Finally, certain paralinguistic behaviors such as attention or defined onset and cessation of motor behavior as the child communicates with desired objects or persons certainly suggests that the action is the means for the child reaching a desired or intended end.

Dyadic actions and shared attention direct the child toward the development of referential meaning in the initial acquisition of grammatical forms. For adult thinkers, action is an abstraction, whereas for the child, action is a tangible form of intended behavior and is a part of the child's incidental learning process. The semantic properties of a verb are acquired in the same interactive process as the semantic characteristics of the noun class. Whatever the adult class, actions, objects, and events remain part of the acquisition of referential meaning. Table 1-2 illustrates how the process of learning an action term parallels the stages of cognitive thinking.

Similar to the agentive and objective referents, the action referents progress very slowly. Specification is made with the emergence of auxiliary verbs and inflectional endings such as -s or -ed or -ing. The verbs are not specified by increasing functional and perceptual attributes associated with the lexical tag as much as they are increased by the way in which the verb may be used with a large number of associated agents, objects, and events. For example, the flexibility of the word "go" is increased by the number of things or people that are related to the action.

Dimensional Referents

Another referent group includes terms that are meaningful in relationship to each other in the same group. The members of this referent group have referen-

Table 1-2 Development of a Referent Illustrating Action

Approximate Age	Adult Question	Child's Response
0-2 Stage 1: Sensory to motor learning	"Shall we go?" "Where shall we go?" "Want to go?" "Are you ready to go?"	Response relates to object or agent moving. The child gets the coat or begins to cry, etc.
2-7 Stage 2: Perceptual and functional attributes are organized through experiences	"What does *go* mean?"	"Well, it's when you go someplace like to the store or it's when you leave for school or when my dog has to go outside, Mom says, 'go.'"
7-11 Stage 3: Concepts are organized and related to experience	"What does *go* mean?"	"Well, it means to leave or when somebody doesn't stay in one place like to move."
11+ Stage 4: Definitions consist of concept complexes	"What does *go* mean?"	"It's a verb that means you aren't staying in the same place but moving from there; it shows action."

tial meaning only because there is another member that can be used to show a relationship. For example, lexical items such as "big" can be understood only when compared to some aspect of the dimension between a size of "bigness" and one of "littleness." The comparison of one member of the class to another member found in the same dimension means that each term has some of the same perceptual semantic features (e.g., E. V. Clark, 1972, 1973, 1974; H. H. Clark, 1973; H. H. Clark & E. V. Clark, 1977).

When one member of the class can be understood only in relationship to another member of the class, the semantic features that separate the meaning of the two words are minimal. This minimal difference usually consists of one semantic feature. Another way of expressing this relationship is to say that when two members of a class are separated by one minimal semantic feature, then the pair is dimensional. The meaning of one of the members of this dimensional relationship is better understood by the speakers, so that each member may be compared to its reference point. In the pair "big-little," the "big" member is in relationship to the "little" member. Thus, "big" would be used in conversation for comparison: "How big is your house?" Linguistically "little" would be considered marked in comparison to the less understood member "big." Seldom would a speaker in this society ask, "How little is your house?" This question would be asked only if the relationship between the two members was shifted by changing the basis of reference. For example: "Houses are small today. I can hardly get enough space to sleep my family." The reference of size now makes "small" or "little" the less understood member. The hearer might now say, "Well, how little is your house?"

It is not always easy to discern the characteristic or semantic feature that separates two members of a dimension. There is a cultural context that establishes the referent of the dimensions for the speakers. In terms of clinical significance, the dimensional terms are in relationship to each other and to the child so that the child needs to practice using the terms in context in order to acquire the semantic features. Learning to label an object in a picture as "big X" or "little X" does not mean that the child is learning the perceptual features necessary to have adult understanding of the concept "big" or "little." Table 1-3 illustrates the theoretical description of dimensional term development for the examples "big" and "little."

The acquisition of these dimensional terms occurs within the first two stages of cognitive thinking. But attaching corresponding ages to the three periods outlined in Table 1-3 is not always accurate since environmental experiences will alter the age of acquisition. With adequate exposure, the size dimensional terms "big" and "little," for example, are usually handled or practiced in conversation by most children three-and-a-half to four years old. These terms are probably easier to learn than some other dimensional terms because they are related more to size than to space.

Table 1-3 Development of a Dimensional Referent

Period I: Sensory to motor learning and attachment of linguistic tags	Big	Child hears the word and may use the word as part of the label, so the child says "big bird" as one word or one concept.
	Little	Again the one-idea term may be used as part of a label for an object, person, or event, as in "little girl."
Period II: Perceptual and functional attributes are organized through experience	Big	The child uses the word for some objects and events. The use may be overexaggerated or overused, and the usage may not be the same as that of an adult. For example, "This is my *big ball*" or "You want *big chair?*"
	Little	The child may overuse this term in place of any dimensional term that has similar characteristics. This also means that one term may be overextended for the other. For example, "little doll" is used when a big relationship is observed by an adult.
Period III: Concepts are organized and related to the appropriate referents		"Big" and "little" are used appropriately and separately in accordance with previous experiences of the dimensional relationship.

Spatial and Temporal Referents

Space and time referents are also learned gradually by a theorized order of complexity. Spatial terms are acquired according to the planes of space and the linguistic markedness of the terms. The three planes of space (horizontal, vertical, and diagonal) correspond to natural referents for a child's growth.

The horizontal position corresponds to the child's early experiences in the supine and prone postures. The horizontal position then yields to the vertical or upright position, separating the child's front from back and left side from right side. The third plane contributes thickness or depth to the child's actions in the horizontal and vertical planes. Consequently, observation and research indicates that the child probably learns the terms denoting the horizontal plane prior to the terms denoting the vertical position. The diagonal plane position is learned last.

Within the referents of space, one member of the pair is more explicit in its informational value and therefore is the linguistically marked member in the specific spatial relationship. For example, within the horizontal plane, "up" and "down" divide some position into an intuitive positive dimension and an intuitive negative dimension. If an adult is sitting at a table, "up" probably would be used to denote anything above the table top, while "down" would be used to denote anything below the table top. This arbitrary division between "upness" and "downness" shifts constantly as the speaker moves from one situation to another. The one constant semantic feature is a horizontal division for all uses of "up" and "down." In some instances there is no way to go but up. For example, an infant on the floor will have an "up" dimension but not a "down" dimension. Since space often extends above the person, it is not surprising that the positive member, "up," is learned first in relationship to the negative member, "down," which is linguistically marked. The marked member is really opposite and the reference point to the member that is used more frequently.

Even though an adult thinker would not believe that these spatial dimensions are referential in nature, the child learns them as concretely as the adult learns new noun vocabulary. Both "up" and "down" are learned because the terms refer to the movements of the child or objects in space. Along the spatial planes, these terms are referential to each other, and adult indication or markings of the terms in an interactive process provides the referential meaning.

The significant point, however, is that the terms develop in relationship to the child. The child's understanding of either term is based on the knowledge the child acquires in space as related to other objects, actions, and events that are being marked by the caretaker in the same space. This incoming information may be altered if the child's input and/or processing skills for spatial relationships are altered. Thus the output regarding the use of these terms would also be different. The difference may reflect the child's inability to associate the lexical term (for example, "up") with the denoted spatial properties. Even if the input is accurate, the association and organization process of the semantic features may be changed, and this alteration would disorganize the way that these spatial terms are utilized.

As the child manipulates and is manipulated within a spatial framework, the terms that denote time are also marked for the child. The child grasps the concept of events that occur simultaneously easier than the concept of events that occur at different times. Therefore, the child first learns the temporal terms that denote immediacy of action, and then gradually learns those temporal pairs that separate time. The acquisition pattern is similar in complexity to that for spatial terms. For most purposes, time has only one dimension that explains a person moving or time moving, a mutually exclusive relationship. Either the person goes through time (as in the utterance, "Next week, I'm going on vacation") or the time moves through the person (as might be expressed by the example, "It's almost two o'clock!"). Table 1-4 illustrates the development of "before" and "after" (E.V. Clark, 1971) as an example of the acquisition of temporal terms.

The gradual learning (from experiences in the environment) of semantic features or information for the terms "before" and "after" occurs during the first two stages of cognitive thinking. Because the acquisition of spatial terms is crucial to the development of temporal terms, these temporal terms will follow an increased understanding of space. A child who has problems with the spatial terms will subsequently have problems with the temporal terms.

The child's acquisition of the dimension of quantity is facilitated by the spatio-temporal acquisition. For example, the term "more" is one of the first words used by a child to request that an action, object, or event be repeated. But the acquisition of "more" (e.g., Donaldson & Balfour, 1968) as in the relationship "more" to "less" is a continual process. Many children in the pri-

---

Table 1-4 Development of Spatial and Temporal Referents

Period I	Before-after	These terms are first learned in the same semantic ways related to space.
	Put the doll in front of the wagon.	The child does this task.
	Later in line— Who was before Susan?	Same interpretation for "in front of."
Period II	Before-after	The terms are confused but "after" is being used.
Period III	Before-after	The terms are more likely to begin to represent time.

mary grades show difficulty with quantity problems such as "Which pile has more beads?"

The referential content of the child's language, including the common classes of adult words—nouns, verbs, adjectives, adverbs, and prepositions—provides the child with lexical terms for expressing all ideas or propositions. The ideas are refined and delineated as the child's experiences with these ideas are increased. Therefore, it is impossible to assess a child's total understanding or comprehension of the stored bits of information. Receptive vocabulary tests or comprehension tests only assess the child's ability to respond to a stimulus (as compared to other children's ability to respond to a stimulus under similar situations). The vocabulary assessment does not reflect the child's active process of semantic acquisition.

COMPREHENSION, PRODUCTION, AND IMITATION

The child's ability to comprehend the previous concepts is an important consideration when dealing with language delayed or disordered children. Axioms such as "receptive language precedes expressive language development" or "the child has to comprehend the words before the child can produce them" have created much confusion in language program development. These kinds of axioms need to be examined both theoretically and therapeutically before accepting them as truths.

The literature regarding children's language comprehension also includes the issues of production and imitation. Based on a review of these studies (e.g., Bloom, Hood, & Lightbown, 1974; Chapman & Miller, 1975; Fraser, Bellugi, & Brown, 1963; Hamilton, 1978; Rees, 1975; Rodd & Braine, 1971; Slobin & Welsh, 1973), this section considers those issues of clinical significance.

Since children's acquisition of the information that underlies the linguistic referents is a gradual semantic and cognitive process, children may very well use a word that is not completely understood. For example the child might say, "My sister has a trike." The adult might ask, "What is a trike?" And the child would respond, "Well, it's a baby bike." Similarly, a child may not respond as an adult would when asked to point to "on the table" or the semantically void stimulus, "point to 'on'. " The child may put things "on" the table in context but may not fully understand all of the semantic perceptual characteristics of that spatial dimension. Therefore, the specific relationships that are represented by the lexical item "on" are not separated from the context. When the child is asked to point to the picture of "on," the child doesn't have a basic relational object or event or action for comparison. A dimensional term without a relationship is limited in referential meaning and therefore limited in its usage.

A child who is asked to say *exactly* what the adult says may be able to imitate longer or more complex sentences than he or she is able to produce in spontaneous conversation. This exact repetition or imitation indicates that production of structural forms may occur before the child actually comprehends those forms. Other examples include the child's ability to recite poems, rhymes, pledges, or songs, or say adult phrases out of appropriate contexts. For instance, consider the following example of a child attempting to use words that are not fully understood.

> Child: "My teacher is a member of the church's new woman's choir."
> Adult: "What does that mean?"
> Child: "Oh, she joined a church that has wire around the outside and new womans are welcome."
> Adult: "What's a new woman?"
> Child: "Maybe she isn't old, maybe she's not married."

The child's extended production under direct imitation does not necessarily equate to the child's linguistic competence. Under spontaneous or elicited imitation situations, the child would change the adult phrase to fit or meet the level of linguistic competence that would match the spontaneous level.

> Adult: "Say what I say: 'The dog is black and white.' "
> Child's Imitation: "The dog is black and white."
> Adult: "Johnny, tell me about the dog that is black and white."
> Child's Spontaneous Response: "The doggie is black and white, too."

When the child's response is elicited from a model but direct imitation is not emphasized, most children will exhibit linguistic patterns that reflect the linguistic competence produced in spontaneous language settings. To the child the form that his or her expression takes is of less importance than the meaning of the utterance.

It should also be noted from the imitation studies that the child's referents stay intact while the older morphemes of modulation are deleted or changed. The wholeness of the basic meaning is evidence of the child's knowledge, and the extent of this knowledge is unclear. The fact that a child may not use a specific inflectional morpheme (for example, -*ing* for present progressive verbs) does not mean the child doesn't understand present progressive activity. For example, "He's going" could be expressed as "He go" or "He go now." Any of the three structures would be meaningful in context, and the adult would understand the child's proposition or idea and intended meaning.

The literature regarding comprehension, imitation, and production is more easily understood if the semantic aspect of the structures is considered. The results might be summarized as follows:

1. Spontaneous use of contentives indicates at least partial knowledge of the lexical item.
2. Spontaneous use of functors indicates at least some linguistic competence in the relationship of that functor to other lexical classes.
3. Elicited or spontaneous imitation is a productive assimilation of another speaker's words to represent the child's ideas.
4. Direct imitation indicates whether or not the child can produce a specific structure, but it does not have a one-to-one correspondence with the child's spontaneous skills.
5. The differences among spontaneous production, elicited imitation, and direct imitation skills are related to the child's comprehension.
6. Comprehension skills are related to responses on a given task as compared to other children on that task, and these skills do not measure a child's total underlying semantic knowledge.

APPLICATION OF THE LITERATURE

From the literature on semantic acquisition as well as from research on imitation, comprehension, and production, it appears evident that a child needs to sensorily receive, process, store, and be able to produce the symbols in order to use language. It is not accurate to assume that the child thinks in sentences before producing basic constructions that are relational and function in a variety of ways. It is not efficient to encourage grammatical adultlike utterances without providing sufficient meaning to support the acquisition of the referents.

Clinical Considerations Regarding Semantics

If a child is having difficulty acquiring the native language, there are several clinical considerations regarding semantic development. The following points summarize the semantic issues most relevant to language intervention.

● The child's language acquisition should reflect development of the basic semantic relations. Children who evidence language disorders often produce or express structural forms that are more complex than those used to express two- and three-term semantic relations. However, when the same language disordered child is requested to reduce these forms to the basic semantic relations, the child's language becomes more spontaneous, indicating a more functional level of development. Thus a child's semantic basis needs to be developed before initiating language programs in which the child is expected to produce adultlike structures.

- Development of a child's comprehension should not be at the expense of the child's learning to use basic semantic relations. The child needs experience using the language to foster more comprehension; referential meaning is acquired by use as well as by passive interaction or experience.

- The child's language experiences at school, home, and in intervention programs should be at the appropriate cognitive level. Language intervention or stimulation should consider the child's level of thinking so that the referential meaning of the tasks is appropriate. For example, an eight-year-old child can't be expected to learn much from a categorization task except the task; the child has not acquired enough semantic features for organization by category.

- Semantic input to the child should be greater than the child's syntactical and morphological levels of development. If the child is in the process of acquiring a language system, then reduction of the linguistic form or structure is better and more natural than reduction of the semantic features in the environment. The adultlike reduction of semantic cues by restriction of experience is more difficult for the child who prefers the semantically rich experience. Furthermore, the cognitive level that corresponds to the semantic level of referential meaning would maximize experiential learning.

- The language materials used in class or in language programs should provide for adequate semantic development. If the child is to acquire the necessary perceptual and functional semantic features, then the materials must also provide exposure to these characteristics. Materials that isolate word meanings from the total concept are too abstract. For example, "night" is a semantic concept that can't be taught by a picture of a boy going to bed. The meaning is limited and the exceptions are not considered; after all, not all people go to bed at night.

- The activities should be selected so that the referents are presented in a variety of ways to build a total concept of a lexical item. Variation of usage fosters the diversity of attributes that constitute a concept. The act of sorting and processing environmental information through usage adds knowledge.

- The activities should be varied so that the contexts provide for language usage and maximum exposure to various semantic relations. For instance, if the child is to compare and contrast incoming information, the child needs opportunities to practice this skill.

- The child's environment should provide ample opportunity to express a variety of intentions. The child's basic intent is to use motor and language skills as a means to an immediate goal. Therefore, if the language is to be used, there must be goals that can be met through that use.

These semantic considerations are of primary importance in developing a program for language delayed or disordered children. If a child has enough semantic development to ignore these considerations, the child's language development will be beyond the basic modulation stages. Thus, corresponding syntactical constructions will be adequately formulated for basic adultlike linguistic communication.

In addition to these, there are also basic considerations that focus on comprehension, production, and imitation. The following principles should be examined prior to planning a language program.

1. If a child learns basic semantic concepts through environmental experiences with the objects, actions, and events that represent the concepts, then the earliest portions of language learning should emphasize production in an environment so that the child has the opportunity to sort the semantic features. This gives the child an opportunity to expand the incoming bits of knowledge. If a child does not produce, it does not mean that the child lacks rudimentary comprehension of basic events. However, the actual linguistic building process may be affected if a child's production is not facilitated. This would imply that a child's comprehension skills may plateau at a lower than expected level if production is not eventful.

2. Imitation is a form of production that may be used to facilitate performance if used at or near the child's level of linguistic competence. This tenet is based on the phenomenon of spontaneous imitation used by most children making the transition from semantic relations expressing basic referents in relationship to one another to modulation of these relations to express more specific referring and predicating. The child may say "Dog go" in context as an "agent + action" relation. This may then be modified to "Dog go bye-bye." This latter utterance is then changed to "The dog go bye-bye," to "The dog is going," and so forth. Most children increase the quantity of verbalization during the period between "Dog go" and "The doggie go bye-bye." This increase is sometimes predominantly by imitation of adults' immediately preceding or past utterances. The utterance (indirect imitation) is reduced to the child's own level of linguistic ability. There is also some exchange of imitation between the parent and the child. The parent says, "Go pick up your blocks," and the child says, "Pick up blocks?" The parent then says, "Yes, go pick up your blocks and put them in the box." Notice that the parent expanded the informational content of the utterance but retained and thus indirectly imitated the main idea.

During this imitation stage of development, the child's increased expression of previously learned and newly learned concepts is incredible. The rising intonation at the end of a parentalreduced utterance will often elicit a spontaneous imitation of the parent's utterance. Therefore, this type of reduction, imitation, and expansion model by the caretaker or other adult is an excellent way to help a child acquire the semantic basis.

3. Direct imitation by the child allows production but not necessarily performance at the child's level of competence. Therefore, direct imitation tasks should be left to those few children who have learned enough of the semantic basis to ignore the basic meaning of the linguistic utterance.

4. The spontaneous and consistent linguistic use of the lexicon is a more accurate indicator than vocabulary tests of a child's comprehension of concepts. The use of the lexicon or vocabulary requires contextual features that govern the spontaneous performance. Therefore, the child's consistent use of vocabulary demonstrates a more complete understanding of the language. Production does not necessarily reflect a one-to-one correspondence with linguistic competence nor comprehension, particularly with language disordered children. Thus a comparison between language comprehension measures and spontaneous production may be a future indicator of what a child might be capable of doing if the production were increased. Conversely, the comprehension measure does not put a limitation on the child's level of production, since production may increase comprehension, further increasing the child's level of production. The child's level of linguistic competence may also be higher than the comprehension measure or production level, thus suggesting that the child's language acquisition is in constant flux.

Although standard measures indicate that levels of comprehension and production are close to the same for normal children, most children with language disorders or delays show a decreased level of complexity in production as compared to that for comprehension. This gap between comprehension and production is additional evidence for justifying the facilitation of production over comprehension in language delayed and disordered children.

SUMMARY OF SEMANTIC DEVELOPMENT AND CLINICAL SIGNIFICANCE

The trends for clinical language intervention in the United States had emphasized the form or construction aspects of an utterance until recent research in early language development signaled the importance of the "meaning" of the words and the relationships of words to the context. As suggested in this first chapter, the development of referential meaning is of primary concern in language intervention because the process of acquiring referents is paramount to a child's development of knowledge from semantic features. The child's referential meaning is a product of a dyadic relationship between the child and others and results in refining changes in language development. While the acquisition of referential meaning allows for the expression of ideas, further expansion of meaning supports linguistic growth in the child's later years. Therefore, the adultlike utterances that develop later are apparently the products of earlier utterances based on the child's intention. Comprehension without production may limit the acquisition of more advanced language-based ideas. Thus adultlike language skills are the product of the interaction between genetic and cognitive abilities and the environmental interaction of language users. Research findings about this process of semantic development provide the requisites for a language assessment intervention strategy suggested in the later chapters. Chapter 2 will describe the semantic rules that govern the use of language skills to meet the child's or speaker's needs.

Practical Questions and Ideas

1. How does a child's level of semantic development influence the materials used in an intervention process?
2. How might the natural techniques of a parent be incorporated into the educator's or clinician's setting?
3. How does a child's level of cognitive processing influence the materials and mode of presentation in a classroom or clinical setting?
4. When does the meaning or content of the language affect the child's performance on imitation, comprehension, or production tasks?
5. What would be the differing variables between a language intervention objective based on facilitating semantic relations and one based on facilitating nouns and verbs?

REFERENCES

Als, H. Social interaction: Dynamic matrix for developing behavioral organization. *New Directions for Child Development*, 1979, *4*, 21-38.

Bates, E., Camaioni, L., & Volterra, V. The acquisition of performatives prior to speech. *Merrill-Palmer Quarterly*, 1975, *21* (3), 205-226.

Berko, J. The child's learning of English morphology. *Word*, 1958, *14*, 150-177.

Bernstein, B. The roles of speech in the development and transmission of culture. In G.J. Klopf & W.A. Hohman (Eds.), *Perspectives on learning*. New York: Mental Health Publishers, 1967.

Bloom, L. *Language development: Form and function in emerging grammars*. Cambridge, Mass.: The MIT Press, 1970.

Bloom, L., Hood, L., & Lightbown, P. Imitation in language development: If, when, and why. *Cognitive Psychology*, 1974, *6*, 380-420.

Bloom, L., Miller, P., & Hood, L. Variation and reduction as aspects of competence in language development. In L. Bloom (Ed.), *Reading in language development*. New York: John Wiley & Sons, 1978.

Bowerman, M. F. Structural relationships in children's utterances: Syntactic or semantic? In T.E. Moore (Ed.), *Cognitive development and the acquisition of language*. New York: Academic Press, 1973.

Bretherton, I., & Bates, E. The emergence of intentional communication. *New Directions for Child Development*, 1979, *4*, 81-100.

Brown, R. The development of wh questions in child speech. *Journal of Verbal Learning and Verbal Behavior*, 1968, *7*, 277-290.

Brown, R. *A first language: The early stages*. Cambridge, Mass.: Harvard University Press, 1973.

Bruner, J. S. Organization of early skilled action. *Child Development*, 1973, *44*, 1-11.

Bruner, J. S. The ontogenesis of speech acts. *Journal of Child Language*, 1974, *2*, 1-19.

Bruner, J. S. From communication to language—A psychological perspective. *Cognition*, 1974-75, *3*, 225-287.

Chapman, R., & Miller, J. Word order in early two and three word utterances: Does production precede comprehension? *Journal of Speech and Hearing Research*, 1975, *18* (2), 355-371.

Clark, E. V. On the acquisition of the meaning of before and after. *Journal of Verbal Learning and Verbal Behavior*, 1971, *10*, 266-275.

Clark, E. V. On the child's acquisition of antonyms in two semantic fields. *Journal of Verbal Learning and Verbal Behavior*, 1972, *11*, 750-758.

Clark, E. V. What's in a word, on a child's acquisition of semantics in his first language. In T. E. Moore (Ed.), *Cognitive development and the acquisition of language*. New York: Academic Press, 1973.

Clark, E. V. Some aspects of the conceptual bases for first language acquisition. In R. L. Schiefelbusch & L. L. Lloyd (Eds.), *Language perspectives, acquisition, and retardation*. Baltimore, Md.: University Park Press, 1974.

Clark, H. H. Space, time, semantics and the child. In T. E. Moore (Ed.), *Cognitive development and the acquisition of language*. New York: Academic Press, 1973.

Clark, H. H., & Clark, E. V. *Psychology and language: An introduction to psycholinguistics*. New York: Harcourt Brace Jovanovich, 1977.

Donaldson, N., & Balfour, G. Less is more: A study of language comprehension in children. *British Journal of Psychology*, 1968, *59*, 461-471.

Ervin-Tripp, S. Some features of early child-adult dialogues. *Language in Society*, 1978, *7*, 357-373.

Foss, D. J., & Hakes, D. T. *Psycholinguistics: An introduction to the psychology of language.* Englewood Cliffs, N.J.: Prentice-Hall, 1978.

Fraser, C., Bellugi, U., & Brown, R. Control of grammar in imitation, comprehension, and production. *Journal of Verbal Learning and Verbal Behavior*, 1963, *2*, 121-135.

Gruber, H. E., & Voneche, J. J. (Eds.). *The essential Piaget.* New York: Basic Books, Inc., 1977.

Hamilton, S. L. *A comparison of the ICP, the TACL, and a spontaneous language sample.* Unpublished master's project, Washington State University, 1978.

Leonard, L. B. *Meaning in child language.* New York: Grune and Stratton, 1976.

Lewis, M., & Brooks-Gunn, J. Toward a theory in social cognition: The development of self. *New Directions for Child Development*, 1979, *4*, 1-19.

Lucas, E. V. The feasibility of speech acts as a language approach for emotionally disturbed children. (Doctoral dissertation, University of Georgia, 1977). *Dissertation Abstracts International*, 1978, *38*, 3479B-3967B. (University Microfilms No. 77-30, 488).

McLean, J., & Snyder-McLean, L. *A transactional approach to early language training.* Columbus, Ohio: Charles E. Merrill, 1978.

Moerk, E. L. *Pragmatic and semantic aspects of early language development.* Baltimore, Md.: University Park Press, 1977.

Moore, T. E. (Ed.) *Cognitive development and the acquisition of language.* New York: Academic Press, 1973.

Nelson, K. Some evidence for the cognitive primacy of categorization and its functional basis. *Merrill-Palmer Quarterly*, 1973, *19*, 21-39.

Ochs, E., & Schieffelin, B. S. (Eds.). *Developmental pragmatics.* New York: Academic Press, 1979.

Olson, D. Language and thought: Aspects of a cognitive theory of semantics. *Psychological Review*, 1970, *77*, 257-73.

Piaget, J. *The language and thought of the child.* New York: World Publishing Co., 1971.

Rees, N. S. Imitation and language development: Issues and clinical implication. *Journal of Speech and Hearing Disorders*, 1975, *40* (3), 339-351.

Rodd, L., & Braine, M. Children's imitation on syntactic constructions as a measure of linguistic competence. *Journal of Verbal Learning and Verbal Behavior*, 1971, *10*, 430-443.

Schlesinger, I. M. Relational concepts underlying language. In R. L. Schiefelbusch & L. L. Lloyd (Eds.), *Language perspectives, acquisition, and retardation.* Baltimore, Md.: University Park Press, 1974.

Sinclair-deZwart, H. Language acquisition and cognitive development. In T. E. Moore (Ed.), *Cognitive development and the acquisition of language.* New York: Academic Press, 1973.

Slobin, D. I., & Welsh, C. A. Elicited imitation as a research tool in developmental psycholinguistics. In C. A. Ferguson & D. I. Slobin (Eds.), *Readings in child language acquisition.* New York: Holt, Reinhart, & Winston, 1973.

Vygotsky, L. S. *Thought and language*. Cambridge, Mass.: MIT Press, 1962. (Originally published, 1934).

Wulbert, M., Inglis, S., Kriegsmann, E., & Mills, B. Language delay and associated mother child interactions. In M. Lahey (Ed.), *Readings in childhood language disorders*. New York: John Wiley & Sons, 1978.

CHAPTER OBJECTIVES

- list and describe the three acts that constitute a speech act according to Searle's description (1969).

- describe the four semantic rules of a speech act.

- explain the four principles of speech acts that may be applied to language therapy settings.

- describe the importance of the four principles of speech acts.

- write the goal of language programs for children who exhibit difficulties using linguistic skills effectively.

- write the rules for one speech act.

- define the terms *pragmatics, illocutionary force indicating devices, primitive speech acts,* and *performatives.*

- explain syntax, morphology, and semantics as each relates to pragmatics.

Chapter 2

Development of a Pragmatic Basis of Language Intervention

Language is akin to the spider's web: The structure is translucent and reproducible, but the irreplicable function is the purpose of its existence.

REVIEW OF THE THEORETICAL BASIS

Chapter 1 considered the development of basic referential meaning and how it helps expand semantic relationships into adultlike sentences. It is necessary to understand semantic development before considering *pragmatics* because pragmatic development refers to the child's acquisition of semantic rules necessary to communicate an intent in order to affect the hearer's attitudes, beliefs, or behavior. This chapter describes the assumed development of the semantic rules within the context of a *speech act,* a theoretical unit of communication between a speaker and a hearer. The speech act, is considered the basic unit of pragmatics here, just as the morpheme is often considered the basic unit of morphology and semantics. The speech act begins its development in the very young child as a prelinguistic and then linguistic social tool. The literature on pragmatics suggests that the social aspect of communication is established through expressed desires and needs that are, more importantly, met. While Chapter 1 focused on the content of the child's linguistic utterances, Chapter 2 focuses on the child's use of this content to meet needs and, especially, to change the environment.

Social Interaction and Language Development

Bruner (1974) suggested that linguistic communication begins in a prelinguistic period during which the child becomes involved in signaling and sequencing rules during play. The rules are part of the semantic development that draws the child's attention to the acts of communication. The rules of interaction are quickly established as the caretaker vocalizes and responds to the infant's coos, smiles, wiggles, and laughs. When the infant vocalizes back to the adult, the caretaker believes that this constitutes a response and so continues to participate in the vocal exchange.

The interaction between the caretaker and the child establishes reciprocal roles—one vocalizes and is the speaker, while the other listens and is the hearer. The roles are then switched. This ability to switch roles is critical to the establishment of a communication process between the child and significant others. In fact, Miller (1978) has developed an approach for establishing turn-taking in language disordered children whom she believes lack social turn-taking skills. Miller suggests that the reciprocal role exchange must be established for functional language to occur.

Consideration as to why some language disordered children do not establish this reciprocal role capacity, is warranted since the answers may suggest an approach for remediation. There are three obvious types of problems that would negatively affect a child's learning of the social, reciprocal roles between speaker and hearer: (1) The child who is sick or has physical limitations may not be able to respond to the caretaker. (2) The child who has processing difficulties may lack appropriate interaction because the semantic basis is inadequate to support social interactions. (3) The child who has difficulty sorting the information of the speaker, or the feedback as a hearer, may show a lack in understanding the semantic rules that govern linguistic interaction. Because reciprocity implies duality, if a child does not respond or initiate as expected, then the caretaker's initiation and response may also change, with the caretaker expecting less in the way of communicative interaction. As parent expectation decreases, then the intention or purposive aspect of social language will also decrease.

Purposive and Intention-Based Linguistic Behavior

Several researchers suggest that the child's prelinguistic and subsequent linguistic acts are intention based and purposive in nature. Halliday (1973, 1975) described two phases of language function observed in his son's early linguistic development. During Phase I, the child, even with limited linguistic skills, showed the ability to express the following functions: *instrumental* (as in "I want"), *regulatory* (as in "do as I tell you"), *interactional* (as expressed by an implied "me and you"), *personal* (as "here I come"), *heuristic* (for curiosity, as might be explained by "tell me why"), *imaginative* (for pretending), and *informative* (to function when the child has something to tell the hearer).

During Phase II, Halliday's child continued to master language functions and moved from the early childlike linguistic utterances to those that more closely resembled adult utterances. Halliday's research is significant in that his child had something meaningful to say based on reasons, functions, or purposes. Furthermore, even a child who is immature linguistically can manipulate a hearer to change the hearer's attitudes, beliefs, or behaviors in some desired direction. In fact, other researchers such as Bates et al. (1975, 1976) suggest that this ability to show purposive behavior for communication is not restricted to linguistic skills but may be observed as early as four months in a child's motor behavior patterns. Certainly a child's attempt to reach for an object, such as a spoon, while vocalizing is an effective form of communication. The adult recognizes this motor act and responds as if the infant had just said, "Please give me the spoon!" Once the infant has been given the object, he or she will often attempt to demonstrate the object's function or indicate the purpose of the request.

The child's intended purpose for performance of the motor and prelinguistic acts appears to establish the function of communicative acts. There has been conflicting literature as to which aspects of early one- or two-term utterances represent semantic relationships and which represent the semantic function. The functions reported by Halliday were sociolinguistic; the function referred to the child's intended purpose to affect the hearer or speaker's environment. Some semantic functions, which usually refer to the purpose of the utterance itself rather than to the intent of the speaker, include: *recurrence* (referent is to reoccur), *nomination* (label of referent), *nonexistence* (absence of referent), *denial* (rejection of referent), *possession* (ownership of referent), and *existence* (presence of referent). Since much of the current literature lists semantic relations and functions together, it is necessary to make some distinction between the sociolinguistic intent (function) of the speaker and the internal purpose of the utterance or its grammatical components (grammatical roles and functions). Unless the word *semantic* appears in front of *function,* function shall refer to the social purpose or intended use of the linguistic act.

If the child demonstrates purposive behavior so that the semantically based utterance has a communicative intent, then the child's ability to express that intention, so as to alter the hearer's attitudes, beliefs, or behaviors, might be considered the child's *communicative competence* (Campbell & Wales, 1970). To know or understand the message of another speaker—that is, to have *linguistic competence* (Chomsky, 1965; Hymes, 1967)—is not enough. *The child must be an active speaker who engages in communicative behavior that is effective at changing the attitudes, beliefs, or behavior of a hearer.*

The child should ideally be able to function as either speaker or hearer in an entire communicative act, including paralinguistic, nonlinguistic, and linguistic features. The speech act encompasses all of these linguistic features as well as the intention of the hearer and the context, purpose, and effects of the linguistic act. The speech act will be the ultimate measure or goal of linguistic ability discussed in this book.

The Speech Act

Austin (1962) explained a speech act as linguistic communication in a process between a speaker and a hearer. The act of doing or performing the speech act accomplished more than the words alone or together could mean. Austin chose to describe this speech act process as consisting of three phases: (1) *locutions;* (2) *illocutions;* and (3) *perlocutions.* Locutionary acts theoretically consisted of the uttering of words plus the proposition or content of the message. Illocutions referred to the performing aspect, such as commanding, promising, and so forth. Perlocutions included the effect of the message on the hearer. Unfortunately, Austin's lack of clarity in describing the requisite conditions of the speech act prohibited the application of his ideas.

Austin's work stimulated much research, but most of the outgrowths were too philosophical or too narrow for communication application. Searle (1969) expanded on Austin's contribution and provided the clarity lacking in Austin's work by suggesting semantic rules for specifying the conditions of a successful speech act. Furthermore, whereas Austin had combined the uttering and the proposition acts, Searle divided these into two separate acts so that the content of the words was not conditionally part of uttering. Therefore, according to Searle, the speech act is composed of the doing aspect *(utterance act),* the meaning component *(propositional act),* and the function *(illocutionary act).* These components will be discussed at length later in this chapter.

The basic tenets of Searle's theory were applied to language disordered children as suggested by Hoag (1975), and then were tested using different populations (Lucas, 1978; Lucas & Hoag, 1976; Mundell & Lucas, 1978). The basic principles of the speech act concept applicable to language therapy include the following:

- Linguistic behavior is *rule governed.*

- Linguistic behavior is the expression of a speaker's *intent.*

- Linguistic behavior is basic to *communication* purposes.

- Linguistic behavior is an *active process.*

According to Searle, all linguistic communication involves linguistic acts. The basic unit of linguistic communication is not the sentence, word, or any symbol, but the *production* of a speech act. Searle (1969) hypothesizes that speaking involves acts such as making statements, giving commands, asking questions, making promises, and so on; and more abstractly, acts such as referring and predicating; and secondly, that these acts are in general made possible by and are performed in accordance with certain rules for the use of linguistic elements. (p. 16)

The literal meaning must be considered for any given context and would include the actual performance of the speech act. Underlying the speech act are the semantic rules specifying the conditions for the particular linguistic devices that determine an utterance as a specific kind of speech act. It is through an explication of the conditions, rules, linguistic devices, and types of speech acts that Searle provides an operational definition of speech acts.

A speech act must have an utterance, a propositional component, and an illocutionary component in order to be complete. However, a speaker may perform an utterance act, a propositional act, and an illocutionary act.

The utterance act occurs when the speaker utters symbols such as morphemes, sentences, and so forth. The propositional act is the primary content of the utterance or the proposition and consists of referring and predicating. Illocutionary acts include those linguistic and paralinguistic indicating devices that determine the force of the proposition. The force is the intent that the proposition is to convey to the hearer. In English, illocutionary force indicating devices include word order, stress, intonation, contour, punctuation, the mood of the verb, plus the so-called performative verbs.

The idea of a *performative* is philosophical at best, but it is an important issue in the development of language. If one word determines the purpose, intent, and basic proposition, then it is a performative. For example, in "I swear . . . " the word "swear" sets the conditions of the utterance so that the hearer presupposes the intent of the message regardless of what follows "swear."

The development of performatives appears to occur prelinguistically. An infant exhibits prelinguistic motor patterns, certain prelinguistic social behaviors that affect a hearer in a certain way. It is assumed that for the child to perform these acts, there must be some preexisting knowledge (see Chapter 1) and some expectations of the context. For example, an adult grabs a child's toy. The child pulls back, throws arms into the air, and gasps. These prelinguistic behaviors are social and communicate an attitude to which the adult responds. Later these prelinguistic behaviors supplement the linguistic skills which are complemented by paralinguistic features. The linguistic utterances are influenced by illocutionary force indicating devices including performative verbs.

The term "marry" is a performative verb that legally unites two people when uttered in the right preexisting conditions. Performative verbs are strong indicators of illocutionary force. Through the speaker's use of these devices, proposition can become a question, a command, a statement, and so forth. Table 2-1 illustrates the development of the system of communication.

Table 2-1 Semantic Development for Communicative Competence

PROPOSITION ACTS

Referents	Predications
Semantic relations	Semantic functions
Conceptual referents	Purpose of functors
a. vocabulary or lexicon	Qualifiers
b. spatio-temporal referents	
c. qualifiers and quantifiers	

LINGUISTIC EXPRESSION—UTTERANCE ACT

Phonology: Rule-ordered acquisition of sound system

Syntax: Integral rule-ordered linerity of word order—
word classes such as nouns, adverbs, verbs, adjectives, conjunctions, articles, prepositions

Morphology: Rule-ordered inflection modulations such as *-s* (third person singular, noun regular plural, possessive)

-*ed* (past regular)

-*ing* (present progressive)

-*ly* (adverb)

-*est* (superlative)

-*er* (comparative)

Rule-ordered morpheme changes such as forms of the copula (to be) for *is, are, been, being, was, were*

forms of modals *(can, will) would, could, should*

forms of negative *don't, can't, won't, shouldn't*

forms of *do* and *does*

forms of *have, has, had*

Phonology, syntax, morphology, interact with and are governed by semantics for a pragmatic system.

Searle divides an effective speech act into the underlying semantic rules that govern the performance of the utterance, proposition, and illocutionary acts. There are two types of semantic rules: regulative and constitutive. *Regulative rules* control preexisting behavior in much the same way as do rules of etiquette. The rule of etiquette that says, "Don't put your elbows on the table" assumes some preexisting conditions which, when present, deter the speaker from placing elbows on the table. The rule, established by the conditions, exists prior to the behavior.

Constitutive rules describe ongoing linguistic activity in much the same ways as the rules that define football, checkers, polkas, chess, and so forth. For example, if the question "What is football?" was posed, the answer would require a description of all of the plays, strategies, and so forth. To play football is to define football by the constitutive rules. Therefore, the process by which the society transmits its culture (Bernstein, 1967) through linguistic means is probably governed by regulative rules. In most cultures a speaker does not turn his or her back to another person because it is not part of the societal conditions. In the context of constitutive rules, speaking with one's back to the hearer is simply not very effective. In terms of application purposes, the constitutive rules are most important since they provide the prerequisites for an effective speech act performance. These rules may define the speech act only as it occurs, like the football game, *not* as a preexisting set of expected behaviors like etiquette regulative rules. A summary statement by Searle suggests

> the semantic structure of a language may be regarded as a conventional realization of a series of sets of underlying constitutive rules, and that speech acts characteristically are performed by uttering expressions in accordance with these sets of constitutive rules. (p. 37)

Constitutive Semantic Rules

The constitutive rules that describe the conditions of a speech act include the *propositional content rule,* the *preparatory rule,* the *sincerity rule,* and the *essential rule.* Each of these rules specifies the linguistic and paralinguistic behaviors that are necessary for the speech act to be effective at affecting the hearer's attitudes, beliefs, or behaviors. The following example illustrates the various parts of the speech act in a format similar to examples presented by Searle.

The illocutionary act is a command; that is, the speaker wishes to affect the behavior of the hearer in a conventional command or rule-order manner. The utterance act is in the sentence form, "Johnny, get the ball!" The underlying semantic rules are as follows:

1. *Propositional content rule.* There is an implied or expected future act (A) of the hearer (H). In this example, "Get (Y) of (X) ball." So the predica-

tion is (Y) of (X) where (X) is the proposition of the function or what is sometimes called the argument (Y). As described in Chapter 1, the mutual experience is attached to the referent "ball" and the expansion or predication about the ball is "get."

2. *Preparatory rule.* There are some understood prerequisites to the utterance.

   a. H is able to do A. The speaker (S) believes H is able to do A.
   b. It is not obvious to both S and H that H will do A in the normal course of events and without some verbal or nonverbal intervention.
   c. S must be in a position of authority at the time of the utterance, since the command effect requires some credibility. In the above example, the speaker must be able to get the ball by using a socially acceptable form of request. The preparatory rule establishes a mutually shared set of conditions that must exist or the linguistic form would not be effective.

3. *Sincerity rule.* Only occasionally in normal speaking situations does the speaker not intend the force of the utterance. That is, only occasionally does the speaker "mean" some force other than the one being communicated. In this example the speaker really does want the ball or the context would become artificial. In the case of jokes, puns, and irony, the sincerity rule is violated. For example: "Get the ball!" "I can't, it's gone!" "I was joking."

4. *Essential rule.* The effect of the intended meaning is realized by the hearer. In the example "Get the ball" the act is not complete until the hearer attempts to get the ball.

The four semantic rules (preparatory, propositional content, sincerity, and essential) are established by the conventions of society. Therefore, a conventional form is understood by other native speakers, and those linguistic devices that determine the type of illocutionary force affect hearers of the language in the same manner.

Application/Speech Acts

Dore (1973) attempted to apply Searle's theory of speech acts to the developmental stages of language acquisition. Dore distinguished between adult speech acts and children's utterances that would have a rudimentary referent (for example, labeling) and a primitive force-indicating device. The primitive speech acts (PSAs) that Dore explained were: labeling, repeating, answering, requesting (answer), requesting (action), calling, greeting, protesting, and practicing. Dore suggested that the child's first utterances do have a function as well as form and that the language may reflect the child's social interactions. Another way to view children who are using one- and two-term semantic relations (just like the ones in Dore's study) is to suggest that the children are attempting to perform an adultlike speech act but do not have all of the components or semantic rules that constitute the adult speech act. For example, the PSA of labeling does not have an adult illocutionary force. In fact, the labeling as defined by Dore may be an adult interpretation of the expression of rudimentary or incomplete components of a speech act. The child says, "Table!" and the parent accepts this as a label. Because the child is ineffective at altering the attitudes, beliefs, or behavior of the hearer, labeling eventually ceases. Since labeling is not apparent in older children, perhaps the assumed function is different from that of labeling. Because the components of the essential rule were rudimentary in labeling; that is, incomplete as compared to the adult prototype, the child's intent is unclear. As the child acquires more advanced linguistic skills the intent is clear. Whereas Dore's labeling, repeating, answering, and practicing lack the referring and predicating constituents for adult speech acts and consequently cease, the other PSAs (calling, greeting, protesting, and requesting) do continue. If the speech act is governed by the semantic rules, a child's PSAs exist because the semantic rules appear to be functioning independently and not together as the rules do in effective or adultlike speech acts.

Whether PSAs are rudimentary or different than the assumed speech acts, four principles of speech act theory that are applicable to language therapy will be discussed as they relate to remediation for the language disordered child. Again, these principles suggest that rule-governed linguistic behavior is the expression of a speaker's intent, is basic to communication purpose, and is an active process.

Rule-Governed Linguistic Behavior

"Speaking a language is engaging in a rule governed form of behavior" (Searle, 1969, p. 22). The constitutive rules of Searle's theory provide the conditions for the performance of a speech act. The essential elements for having a particular effect on a hearer can then be specified according to the illocutionary indicating devices. If a child experiences difficulty with acquiring or using these rules and with the specifications of these rules, then the child would evidence a pragmatic language problem. From this theoretical basis, then, a pragmatic language problem has its basis in semantics.

In this section the rules are described for eight speech acts selected from the literature that relates speech acts to normal children's language acquisition (Bruner, 1974; Dore, 1974a, 1974b); from clinical observations of the needs of language disordered children (Lucas & Hoag, 1976; Lucas, 1977); from the theoretical literature on sociolinguistics and the philosophy of language (Searle, 1969; Halliday, 1975); from child language acquisition data (e.g., Bloom,

1970; Brown, 1973); and from therapy intervention literature now available about semantics and pragmatics (McLean & Snyder-McLean, 1978; Schiefelbusch, 1978). The eight speech acts include requests for objects, requests for actions, assertions, denials, statements of information, requests for information, callings or summons, and rule orders. Other speech acts such as reports or experiences are really speech events, much like the task of "describing" consists of a series of speech acts.

The eight selected speech acts may be defined in a fashion similar to specifications given for examples of speech acts (Searle, 1969):

1. *Requests for Objects* (similar to requests. Searle, 1969, p. 66*)

Propositional Content Rule:	Future act A of H.
Preparatory Rule:	1. H is able to provide A. S believes H knows what A is and that H has A.
	2. It is not obvious to both S and H that H will provide A in the normal course of events of his own accord.
Sincerity Rule:	S wants H to do A.
Essential Rule:	Counts as an attempt to get H to do A.

The following elements are included as a necessary part of the essential rule for the H to be appropriately affected:

1. S's body orientation is toward H in order to ready H for the utterance.
2. Eye contact or name is used to signal H.
3. Appropriate linguistic markers indicating either
   a. an interrogative form
   b. an imperative form.
4. An utterance which specifies what H is to do.
5. Appropriate loudness for H to respond.

2. *Requests for Action*

Propositional Content Rule:	Future act A of H.
Preparatory Rule:	1. H is able to do A. S believes H is able to do A.
	2. It is not obvious to both S and H that H will do A in the normal course of events of his own accord.
Sincerity Rule:	S wants H to do A.
Essential Rule:	Counts as an attempt to get H to do A.

---

* This adaptation by permission of J. R. Searle.

The following elements are included as a necessary part of the essential rule:

1. S's body orientation is toward H in order to ready H for the utterance.
2. Eye contact or name used to signal H.
3. Appropriate linguistic markers indicating either:
   a. an interrogative form
   b. an imperative form.
4. An utterance which specifies what H is to do.
5. Appropriate loudness for H to respond.

3. *Assertion*

Propositional Rule:	Any proposition p.
Preparatory Rule:	1. S has evidence (reason, etc.) for the truth of p.
	2. It is not obvious to both S and H that H knows (does not need to be reminded of, etc.) p.
Sincerity Rule:	S believes p.
Essential Rule:	Counts as an undertaking to the effect that p represents an actual state of affairs.

The following elements are included as a necessary part of the essential rule for the utterance of an assertion:

1. A falling contour representative of a declarative form.
2. A form of ___ is X, which does not follow by direct imitation, is used (otherwise S would know that H is already aware of p).
3. The utterance is given with appropriate loudness.
4. Eye contact is given to signal H, or observation is given to signal H.
5. Body orientation between S and H within a front plane position.

4. *Denial*

Propositional Rule:	Past act A done by H is in the p form of not X.
Preparatory Rule:	1. S does not believe that it is in his better interest to do as X indicates.
	2. The p is obvious to both H and S.
Sincerity Rule:	S does not want to do X.
Essential Rule:	Counts as an attempt to deny H's p.

The following elements are considered part of the essential rule for a denial:

1. The previous action or p of the H is implied through gesture or is linguistically specified.
2. Use of emphatic stress or loudness for H to respond.

3. The utterance is negatively marked.
4. Eye contact is used to signal H.
5. Orientation is toward H or toward the action or materials being denied.

5. *Statements of Information* (differs from Searle's assertion)

Propositional Rule:	Any proposition p.
Preparatory Rule:	1. S knows of p to be fact or evidence of fact.
	2. It is not obvious to H what p is. In fact, it is obvious to S that H does not know p.
Sincerity Rule:	S believes that H needs the information and cannot get the information elsewhere.
Essential Rule:	Counts as an attempt to state the information.

The following elements are included as part of the essential rule:
1. A falling contour representative of a declarative form.
2. Appropriate loudness for H to respond.
3. Content is factual for H.
4. Eye contact signals H, or observation signals H.
5. Orientation of the body is toward H.

6. *Requests for Information*

Propositional Content Rule:	Future act A of H.
Preparatory Rule:	1. S believes H knows X (p) and H is able to tell S.
	2. It is not obvious that S will find out without asking H.
Sincerity Rule:	S wants H to tell X (p).
Essential Rule:	Counts as an attempt to get H to tell (p).

The following elements are included as part of the essential rule for requests for information:
1. The utterance is marked with a rising contour.
2. The utterance utilizes a specific lexical item indicating a constituent question or an interrogative reversal indicating the answer to a yes/no question.
3. Appropriate loudness is used for H to respond.
4. Eye contact signals H or observation signals H.
5. Body orientation is either toward the materials or toward H.

7. *Calling or Summons:*

Propositional Content Rule:	Future act A of H.
Preparatory Rule:	1. S believes that H will not notice or do A without S telling him.
Sincerity Rule:	S wants H to do A.
Essential Rule:	Counts as an attempt for S to get H.

The following elements are considered as part of the essential rule:
1. The H is specified by name or is signalled by some other linguistic marker of notification.
2. Orientation is facing H.
3. Eye contact or observation is made during or as a part of the utterance.
4. The utterance specifies how H is to perform or respond.
5. The loudness is adequate for H to respond.

8. *Rule Orders*

Propositional Content Rule:	Future act A of H.
Preparatory Rule:	1. S believes that H does not know the rule of the situation.
	2. S does not think H will know it unless he tells him.
Sincerity Rule:	S believes that H should know rule.
Essential Rule:	Counts as an attempt for S to understand H.

The following elements are considered as part of the essential rule:
1. The utterance is given with a falling contour for an imperative form.
2. The utterance is given with adequate loudness for H to respond.
3. Body orientation is toward H.
4. Eye contact signals H, or observation signals H.
5. The utterance specifies what H is to do.

By describing these eight speech acts according to their underlying semantic rules, the part of the speech act that is difficult for the child may be determined, analyzed, and facilitated. The use of the speech act for planning intervention will be explained in more detail in later sections.

Intention-Based Linguistic Behavior

Although a child's language may be rule-governed as explained previously in this chapter, unless the child has specific ideas or intentions to express, the language will seem meaningless and probably won't be used to alter the attitudes, beliefs, or behaviors of hearers. Figure 2-1 illustrates the speech act as it is sub-

Figure 2-1 Components of the Speech Act: A Linguistic Process of Communication

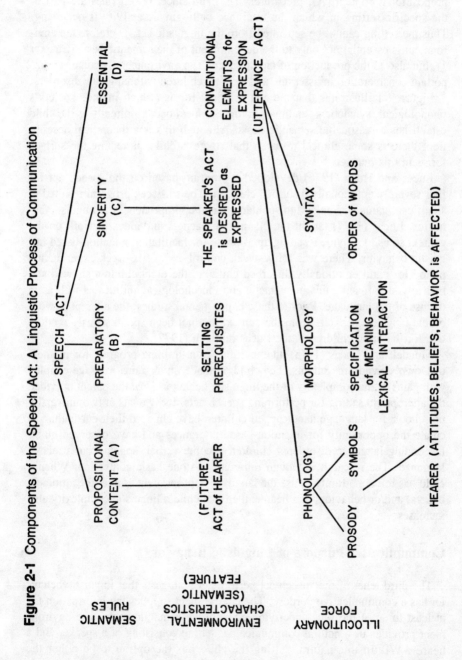

divided into the semantic rules and their corresponding surface structures. The propositional content (A), preparatory (B), and sincerity (C) rules are part of the specific setting in which the utterance or linguistic activity is occurring. Thus the setting cannot be separated from the linguistic act. Therefore the environment is essential not only to the development of the semantic basis (Chapter 1), but also to the production of an utterance. The environment becomes an important consideration in assessing and treating children with language disorders.

Figure 2-1 illustrates that the conventional forms (which include society's phonological, syntactical, and morphological rules) occur indirectly as the child establishes a reasonable semantic basis. Although this is a theoretical description, there is some clinical research that suggests children acquire the surface forms in this manner.

Lucas and Hoag (1976) developed a program based on the speech act for four severely emotionally disturbed children. The six-week program resulted in significant gains with regard to spontaneity and appropriateness of linguistic behavior. Lucas (1977) taught the classroom teachers and aides to work on the context so as to provide a setting appropriate for facilitating intention-based linguistic behavior. There was a five-week control and a five-week experimental period for eight emotionally disturbed children; the eight children showed statistically significant gains in syntactic and morphological abilities as well as in the use of the language. Prior to these experimental studies, the attempt to work on the language separate from the context had not been spontaneously productive for the eight children in the Lucas research (1977).

Mundell and Lucas (1978) attempted a parent-training program for mothers of Down's Syndrome infants. The children made quick gains in usage coupled with gains in the complexity of the linguistic behavior *when* the parent provided the appropriate setting for performing speech acts. Individuals at two university preschools for language handicapped children have changed their curriculum to create the opportunity for intention-based utterances and have observed quiet, responding language disordered children become verbal, spontaneous users of language. The research, although minimal, has one basic contention: When a child has the opportunity to use the language appropriately to alter the attitudes, beliefs, and/or behaviors of a hearer, then that child's linguistic complexity also increases.

Communicative Purpose of Linguistic Behavior

The third tenet of the speech act performance suggests that linguistic behavior has a communicative purpose. The environment supplies the information for at least three of the four underlying constitutive semantic rules. The environment provides us a natural communicative setting consisting of a speaker and a hearer. Within this natural setting the child has the option to be either the speaker or the hearer. By exchanging roles the child has the chance to practice expressing intentions and learns the binding forces between the self and the others in the environment. The resulting social interactions illustrate the communicative purpose that underlies linguistic behavior. As suggested in Chapter 1, the opportunity to change roles in social interactions appears to change the linguistic productivity.

Active Process of Linguistic Behavior

The total concept of the speech act is that it involves a performance in a context according to society's rules. The child must perform as an active participant in the environment. The child who merely responds to productions that someone else makes (either through imitation and/or through tasks of speaking that are not attached to meaningful environmental aspects), is not performing speech acts and consequently is not using language. Active involvement in the situation is critical to becoming an effective speaker and hearer. From Searle's (1969) explanation of speech acts: "A theory of language is part of a theory of action . . . ." (p. 17). A child who produces an utterance according to the rules that include contextual rules is producing or attempting to produce a speech act.

PRAGMATICS: APPLICATION OF THE LITERATURE

The child who exhibits a pragmatic problem has difficulty being effective in altering the attitudes, beliefs, and/or behaviors of a hearer. This same child is by definition also experiencing difficulty in acquiring the semantic rules that govern the use of linguistic and paralinguistic skills for communication. The general disruption may occur in any of these four areas: (1) developing the rules; (2) establishing a desire or motivational cause for having an intent to linguistically express; (3) having a need to communicate to a hearer; and/or (4) being capable of participating in the active process. Each of these principles of the speech act is discussed in the next section.

Acquiring the Semantic Rules

As explained in Chapter 1, establishing referential meaning (propositional rule) with the child's significant others is crucial to language development. However, as delineated in the specifications for the eight common speech acts, the child must be able to understand the preparatory and sincerity conditions of the context. The essential components are acquired through environmental models; the child who acquires these is capable of participating as a performer as well as a hearer.

From clinical experience it is apparent that some children do not have the social ability to differentiate or to change their own behaviors. For example, while most children face a hearer while speaking, some children begin to speak while performing in ways that do not allow the hearer to be readied for the proposition. Consequently, the child does not affect the hearer in the desired manner. This lack of effectiveness only adds to the negative value the child places on the communicative task. When the child is taught to signal the hearer by raising the hand or tugging at the hearer's shirt, the child is much more successful and the communicative task takes on positive value.

What causes these unusual patterns of communication may be related in some instances to the overall behavioral symptoms of the emotionally disturbed child; but facilitating pragmatic language often reduces the behavioral symptoms that were initially used as part of the diagnosis. Thus the diagnosis and symptoms are the same entity. Furthermore establishing a special education diagnosis is not always a means of detecting children with pragmatic problems since children who are reticent, verbally aggressive, or nonverbal also may have some problems with one or more aspects of the semantic rules.

The use of the conventional symbols is established under the essential rule components. So syntax, phonology, and morphology must also be simply intact at the level of complexity necessary to refer and/or predicate. As described in Chapter 3, disorders of the semantic rules result in some characteristic symptoms that may be analyzed qualitatively (Chapter 4) and planned for in remediation.

Motivational Experience

Although ideas may be acquired through passive environmental manipulation, the intent to communicate the idea is a dynamic process existing between the speaker and the environmental conditions.

In order for the child to produce an intention-based utterance, there must be a desire. In other words the child must have a desire that requires linguistic recognition to be met by external changes. If the environmental conditions make it unnecessary that the child use linguistic skills, speech acts will not be performed. Likewise, the motivational values of situations and objects vary among children according to social maturity. Chapter 8 will suggest techniques for establishing the opportunity or need to use linguistic skills in an intentional, purposive manner.

Communication Value

In order for the child to experience positive communication, the hearers in the child's environment must be consistent and supportive. If hearers ignore the child's communication attempts, if the feedback from the child's internal or external systems is confusing, and/or if the environment responds negatively to communication attempts; the value of any communication attempt is lessened for the child. Thus, the likelihood of the child's attempting to perform speech acts decreases.

Participation in the Active Process

A speech act is not complete or performed unless all of the critical components are included. Therefore the child who is seldom in the position to perform a speech act is seldom going to be an effective communicator. Since production of the semantic aspects results in increased language development (Chapter 1), and because clinical evidence suggests that more effective communication increases language productivity (Lucas, 1977), the language disordered child should be guided through the performance of successful speech acts. A goal of language programs for children with pragmatic language disorders would be the successful completion of speech acts. Only when the child actually performs speech acts, does the child become part of the active process.

SUMMARY OF PRAGMATIC APPLICATION

The form of language is complex but easily discernible. Its purpose rests with the speaker's ability to express an intent for altering a hearer's attitudes, beliefs, or behavior. Thus, the semantic rules (which are a theoretical explanation of a speech act) are developed through use, feedback, and refinement of the essential components. These rules may be used as the criteria against which one can judge a normal speaker's ability to communicate effectively. Consequently, a child suspected of exhibiting a language disorder may be compared against the normal speaker's performance to determine the areas of pragmatic weakness. Chapter 3 will describe the possible disorders that stem from semantic problems and result in communicator ineffectiveness and/or inefficiency.

Questions

1. Why was the speech act chosen as the unit for studying pragmatics?
2. What effects does the environment have on language usage?
3. How does the speech act unit apply to language intervention?
4. What is the purpose of using a theoretical construct for a basis to language intervention?
5. Why is ineffectual communication actually a semantic language problem?

REFERENCES

Austin, J. L. *How to do things with words*. London: Oxford University Press, 1962.

Bates, E. Pragmatics and sociolinguistics in child language. In D. M. Morehead & A. E. Morehead (Eds.), *Normal and deficient child language*. Baltimore, Md.: University Park Press, 1976.

Bates, E., Camaioni, L. & Volterra, V. The acquisition of performatives prior to speech. *Merrill-Palmer Quarterly*, 1975, *21* (3), 205-226.

Bernstein, B. The role of speech in the development and transmission of culture. In G. J. Klopf & W. A. Hohman (Eds.), *Perspectives on learning*. New York: Mental Health Publishers, 1967.

Bloom, L. *Language development: Form and function in emerging grammars*. Cambridge, Mass.: The MIT Press, 1970.

Brown, R. *A first language: The early stages*. Cambridge, Mass.: Harvard University Press, 1973.

Bruner, J. S. The ontogenesis of speech acts. *Journal of Child Language*, 1974, *2*, 1-19.

Campbell, R., & Wales, R. The study of language acquisition. In J. Lyons (Ed.), *New horizons in linguistics*. Harmondsworth: Penguin, 1970.

Chomsky, N. *Aspects of the theory of syntax*. The Hague: Mouton, 1965.

Dore, J. The development of speech acts (Doctoral dissertation, City University of New York, 1973). *Dissertation Abstracts International*, 1973, *34*. (University Microfilms No. 73-14, 374.)

Dore, J. A pragmatic description of early language development. *Journal of Psycholinguistic Research*, 1974, *3* (4) 343-350. (a)

Dore, J. Holophrases, speech acts, and language universals. *Journal of Child Language*, 1974, *2*, 21-40. (b)

Halliday, M. A. K. *Explorations in the functions of language*. New York: Elsevier North Holland, 1973.

Halliday, M. A. K. *Learning how to mean: Explorations in the development of language*. New York: Elsevier North Holland, 1975.

Hoag, L. *Application of speech act theory to language disordered children: The program*. Unpublished manuscript, University of Illinois, 1975.

Hymes, D. H. Models of interaction of language and social setting. *Journal of Social Issues*, 1967, *23*, 8-28.

Lucas, E. V. The feasibility of speech acts as a language approach for emotionally disturbed children (Doctoral dissertation, University of Georgia, 1977). *Dissertation Abstracts International*, 1978, *38*, 3479B-3967B. (University Microfilms No. 77-30, 488.)

Lucas E., & Hoag, L. *Speech acts: A language therapy strategy for emotionally disturbed children.* Paper presented at the Interdisciplinary Linguistics Conference: Language Perspectives, Louisville, Kentucky, May 1976.

McLean, J., & Snyder-McLean, L. *A transactional approach to early language training.* Columbus, Ohio: Charles E. Merrill, 1978.

Miller, L. *Pragmatics: An assessment/intervention model used with an autistic child.* Paper presented at the American Speech and Hearing Association, San Francisco, November 1978.

Mundell, C., & Lucas, E. *A parent conducted pragmatic language program for Down's Syndrome children.* An unpublished manuscript, Washington State University, 1978.

Schiefelbusch, R. L. (Ed.). *Language intervention strategies.* Baltimore, Md.: University Park Press, 1978.

Searle, J. R. *Speech acts: An essay in the philosophy of language.* Cambridge, England: Cambridge University Press, 1969.

CHAPTER OBJECTIVES

- list various semantically based language disorders.

- describe the characteristics of the semantic disorders.

- explain the relationship between the semantic disorders and the child's pragmatic difficulties.

- describe the differences between a language delay and a language disorder.

- give language sample examples for each type of semantic language disorder.

- demonstrate the relationship between the speech event, the speech act, and the described disorders.

- explain the rationale for determining specific language disorders.

- explain the relationship between specific language disorders and a general language delay.

- explain the relationship between language development and those language disorders with a semantic basis.

- explain the characteristics of each of the language disorders.

Chapter 3

Descriptions of Semantic and Pragmatic Language Disorders

The balance of a personality rests delicately between its social projections and its meaningful presence; disrupt the purpose and malady is inevitable.

LANGUAGE DELAY VERSUS LANGUAGE DISORDER

The child's ability to communicate socially may be impaired in three basic ways:

1. The child may not adequately acquire the perceptual and functional characteristics of objects, actions, and/or events, therefore restricting the semantic referential basis.
2. The child may not be able to relate the lexicon with the objects, actions, and/or events, so that the semantic basis for further language development is limited.
3. The child may not systematically acquire the semantic rules underlying the speech act described in Chapter 2.

If any of these problems occur, singly or in combination, then the child will eventually manifest a general or specific language disorder.

At this point it is important to understand what constitutes a language delay as opposed to a general or specific language disorder. A *language delay* is manifested by the interruption of language development, even though the presently acquired language maintains its systematic and sequential characteristics. Systematicity of language refers to the usual organized acquisition of specific skills; the skills emerge one by one or in a sequential pattern similar to other children at the same level of development. A delay is usually most apparent in the child's syntax and acquired morphological rules, because these show up on

51

the surface. When there is a delay in the child's semantic development, it generally affects the language structures, so determination of semantic problems is more difficult. When semantic errors automatically disrupt the mapping on of structures, then the child no longer has a systematic or sequential language acquisition.

When the language acquisition is not systematic and/or sequential, semantic errors must be considered the symptoms of a *language disorder*. The number and type of semantic errors determine whether there is a disorder in a specific area of linguistic development or whether the disorder will affect various linguistic skills and consequently be considered a general language disorder. For example, when a child experiences difficulty with the concepts related to space and time, this constitutes a specific language disorder. Or a child may experience difficulty in many areas of semantic development, resulting in an overall communication problem that affects both academic and social development. Since pragmatic language is based on semantic development, a child who has difficulty in using the language really has a disorder in semantic development.

An example will illustrate the differences between a delayed language child and a disordered language child. The following segments of language were collected from two four-year-old children who exhibit similar structural levels of linguistic development; that is, each child has a comparable mean length of utterance (MLU) calculated on a minimum of 50 utterances. Brown's (1973) description of determining an MLU was used for the calculation.

Child A, Male (MLU = 4.8)	*Child B, Male* (MLU = 4.9)
1. Keep the truck!	1. Give me that, please.
2. I'm going to see Charlie.	2. I have that.
3. Charlie, let's play on the swing.	3. No more glue, please.
4. You be the rider and I be the pilot.	4. I don't have any of that yellow glue, see?
5. Come on!	5. See, I need more yellow glue.
6. Let's go.	6. When did you go?
7. Charlie, you be the rider.	7. Where do you live?
8. Up, up, and away! Varoom!	8. Do you have a house?
9. All right, everyone out!	9. What is your name?
10. Jump, the plane is on fire.	10. Jimmy.

These utterances were taken from a representative portion of the language sample and were produced consecutively. The clinician's responses were following comments that did not lead the child in any obvious way. Whether or not the utterances are quantitatively calculated, that is, whether or not numerical calculations such as an MLU are determined, the quality of each utterance should be evaluated. The evaluation of quality should consider: (1) How well does the child use the semantic rules to affect a hearer? (2) Are the utterances truly part of the context? (3) Are the utterances typical of a child this age? and (4) Do the utterances flow smoothly in content and ideation?

The differences in quality between the language of Child A and Child B should become apparent as the questions are answered. (Chapter 4 will expand on the qualitative analysis of a language sample.) For now, the distinction between a delay and disorder is basically determined by Child A's ability to use the language and Child B's inability to use the semantic rules. Child B does have a moderate pragmatic language disorder even though his sentence structure is good. Child A has some age-related problems with morphophonemic rules (for example, "be" is used for the future construction), but Child A's intent is clear as indicated by the use of semantic rules requiring the referential meaning to be clear.

To further explain the distinction between a delay and disorder, the same utterances will be considered with the adult's utterances put into the context. From a pragmatic perspective, the context is important in assessing communicative competence.

	Child A		*Child B*
1.	Keep the truck! *Adult:* Why do you want me to keep the truck?	1.	Give me that, please. Which one do you want?
2.	I'm going to see Charlie. *Adult:* Okay.	2.	I have that. What do you have?
3.	Charlie, let's play on the swing. (No adult comment)	3.	No more glue, please. Okay, I have the glue.
4.	You be the rider and I be the pilot. *Charlie:* "Okay, sure."	4.	I don't have any of that yellow glue, see? Yes, I see.
5.	Come on! (Charlie is looking at the grass.)	5.	See, I need more yellow glue. Yes, I see that you need more yellow glue.
6.	Let's go. (Tugs on Charlie.) (Charlie goes with Child A.)	6.	When did you go? What do you mean?
7.	Charlie, you be the rider. Okay, quit pushing.	7.	Where do you live? In Jonesborough.
8.	Up, up, and away! Varoom! Come on, recess is over.	8.	Do you have a house? Well, I do own my house.
9.	All right, everyone out! (Child A pulls the swings sideways.)	9.	What is your name? You know what my name is!
10.	Jump, the plane is on fire. (Child A and Charlie run to the door.)	10.	Jimmy. No, that is your name.

Given the context of the others' utterances, plus a little information on the present activities, it is apparent that Child B has many semantic/pragmatic difficulties. For example, following the referent of the conversation as well as following the referent of the tasks are problems. Also notice that in Child B's fourth and fifth utterances, the intent was probably different than indicated by the linguistic skills. Child B is actually asking the adult for more yellow glue, but instead asks the adult if she sees the yellow glue and if she sees that he doesn't have any glue. Child B never asks the teacher for the glue. Furthermore, in the third utterance Child B says he doesn't want any more glue. This is also inaccurate information because Child B doesn't have any glue at the time. The adult's comment was really a confirmation that he couldn't have any more glue so long as the adult had it.

Closer examination of Child A's utterances shows that this child is capable of following the referent in the environment and the topic of conversation. He shows the ability to affect the hearer's behavior, whereas Child B was showing great difficulty in modifying or influencing the hearer. Since Child A's language appears to be semantically intact and pragmatically effective, this child's structure must be considered. Structurally, Child A is slightly delayed according to what might be expected for a child of his age. But Child B is disordered regardless of his chronological age. The primary distinction between Child A and Child B, based on these few utterances, is that Child A is capable of producing utterances that relate directly to the conversation or present topic, whereas Child B is not capable of following the situational referent in order to produce utterances that may modify the setting. In other words, Child B is ineffective at conveying his intent to a hearer because of semantic difficulties.

The distinction between language delay and disorder will be expanded in later chapters. For now, an operational definition is presented: a language delayed child is progressing systematically and sequentially in all aspects of linguistic development including appropriate usage. A language disordered child is not progressing systematically and sequentially in any aspect of rule-governed and purposive linguistic behavior.

Since semantic errors greatly influence the disordered language production and often create a pragmatic problem, the specific semantic errors will be discussed individually. Although specific semantic errors may only affect communication, they more often affect the child's academic development as well. The terminology used to describe semantic errors is based on the symptoms and in some cases on previous literature.

SPECIFIC SEMANTIC DISORDERS

Auditory Misperception

An *auditory misperception* is manifested by specific sound confusions, and when frequently produced is found with other semantic difficulties related to the child's semantic sequencing. *Semantic sequencing* refers to the ability to organize actions, objects, and/or events according to the linguistic knowledge ascribed to these items. There is a linearity of linguistic order for the language, but sequencing in this instance refers to the ability to relate the semantic concepts. English linearity, which is governed primarily by word order, will be discussed under the syntactic problems.

This problem of specific sound confusions was labeled auditory misperception because the child who exhibits this difficulty does not appear to auditorily recognize the errors being made in the specific words. Examples of auditory misperceptions collected from children's language samples include the following consistent errors: "bressed" for "dressed"; "dreakfast" for "breakfast"; "pant" for "plant."

If children with auditory misperceptions were given an articulation test (incidentally, any of the children used as examples in this chapter have been given complete diagnostic batteries, including articulation assessment), the errors of the type found in the "bressed" for "dressed" confusion would usually not appear on the test because the child's production has little to do with the error patterns. Furthermore, the child with auditory misperceptions may or may not do well on an auditory discrimination test involving choices between rhyming words or rhyming nonsense syllables. Most of the children who exhibit auditory misperceptions do in fact score poorly on batteries of auditory perception and discrimination tests. Unfortunately, the converse relationship has not been noticed. Not all children who do poorly on auditory discrimination and/or perception tests evidence auditory misperceptions. When these errors occur periodically, they are usually considered slips of the tongue. A child who evidences a periodic misperception coupled with any academic difficulty should be assessed for a possible general language disorder. Although auditory misperceptions occur as seldom as once or twice in every 100 spontaneous utterances, they are a clue to the child's overall language intactness.

The presence of auditory misperceptions is an indication of a more general language problem. As will be discussed later, the clinician's primary emphasis will not be on auditory misperceptions but on the overall language problem.

Off Target Responding

When a child says something that does not fit the adult's expectation as to what is appropriate in that situation, the adult might say that the child is "out to lunch," a "space cadet," a little "spacey," or maybe "off the wall." A child who is off target in responding is not able to scan the previous utterances or the surrounding context for appropriate referent possibilities. If the child cannot determine the referent, then the utterance(s) may be referentially off the target idea in responding.

The word "responding" is used to denote that the child is part of a speaker-to-hearer paradigm in which the child is listening, while speaking, and thus monitoring her or his own utterances. The child is also hearing and monitoring what the other speaker is saying. Therefore, if the child is listening as a hearer and is attending to the environmental contextual cues, the child is responding to all sets of information. The child's response should indicate that the child has successfully recognized the important cues and can use those cues to maintain the topic of conversation by referring to the referent and by commenting or predicating something about the referent.

The child who is not able to respond on target is experiencing difficulty with processing and/or attaching the sign to the symbol. For example, the word "cat" is the visual sign for an animal that is characterized and subsequently recognized by its functional and perceptual attributes (a cuddly, furry creature with four legs and a characteristic "meow"). The symbol is the representation of the perceptual and functional attributes. In other words, to distinguish a "cat" from a "dog" requires an ability to distinguish among these characteristics.

If the child's perception of the environment is different from others' perceptions, then the child will process the symbols differently and subsequently attach the signs differently. The etiology for such an inability is at best hypothesized: possibly the child is emotionally disturbed or mentally retarded; perhaps the child has perceptual difficulties; perhaps the child has an acuity difficulty that results in the child seeing a partial image which is then attached with an unusual sign. Whatever the etiology, the linguistic symptoms are the same.

Off target and off topic responding occurs when the referent is not the one expected in that context. The errors increase in frequency as the child's knowledge and expected linguistic skills become more complex. For example, the child who is experiencing difficulty in staying on topic will show more errors as constituent questions or the corresponding answers become more complex. The question, "What is that?" is relatively simple because the constituent "what" refers to an object (symbol) that is acquired as an early semantic relation. The naming game (that is, "What that?" = "That what!") is part of the deixis assumed in the infant's roles with the caretakers. Therefore, "What is that?" is a simple question to answer linguistically if the child has the knowledge.

If an older child can't answer the same question because of lack of experience with the subject, then the older child will say, "I don't know" or ask for some kind of clarification. The child who has trouble staying on topic will respond with an answer to some other question not yet asked. For example, an older language disordered child may respond to "Johnny, what's that?" with "I did my homework, Ms. Smith."

The language disordered child may develop the basic semantic relations and the appropriate structure, but an understanding of social implications is not always apparent. The child will experience more difficulty as questions and referents become more advanced, requiring inferences and conclusions about invisible objects or actions, and events no longer present. Off target utterances may also occur in conversations in which the referent is removed, therefore increasing the difficulty. The presence of a referent as in the example "What is that?" makes the question easier.

The following segment of off target utterances were taken from a child in a special classroom:

"John, please take your work folder out of your desk."
"I can't find my math paper, Ms. Smith."
"John, you turned your math paper in to me yesterday."
"Well, I can't find my paper . . . the one with the math on it."
"John, listen to me. You turned your math paper in to me."
"Ms. Smith, I got to find my math paper. It isn't in my work folder."

The child is not processing the referential meaning of Ms. Smith's utterances. The child is off target and off topic.

The following segment is from a therapy session in which the clinician is working with an adolescent Down's Syndrome client:

"Mary Lou, did you have a party?"
"Yes, had one downstairs."
"Is the party over?" (The time referential use of "over" is difficult.)
"See, my new dress."

The dress isn't new, but the switch in topic is Mary Lou's device for not answering a question that is too difficult. Mary Lou is no longer on topic.

The following segment is from a seven-year-old learning disabled child enrolled in a resource room for part of the day:

"What did you have for lunch?" ("What" is a simple referent and the question is one that has probably been asked before.)
"I had a sandwich and a banana."
"Anything else?"
"No, I don't think so."
"What does your Dad do?" (The referent of the utterance is literally *"Dad do"* but the referential meaning is removed.)
"He sleeps a lot, well, I mean, when he paints around."
"Does your Dad paint?" (Even though this is a simple is/does ques-

tion requiring a yes/no answer, the child is capable of recognizing
the implied question about what kind of painting, etc.)
"Well, sometimes he paints, and you see, he works all around the
school building, painting or something alike this, well . . . my Dad
owns a motorcycle."

From the last utterance, it appears that it is easier for this child to change
topics when it is his turn to speak than to try to adjust his utterances to the appropriate topic. Obviously this child has the knowledge but not the ability to
use the necessary linguistic skills to convey the message that he intends. The
same child does beautifully on listening to a long paragraph and answering a
choice question requiring some kind of conclusions. The inferences and conclusions are always retrievable even though the manner of expression is poor.

In the three language samples presented, each of the children was differen-
tially diagnosed but exhibited the same off target problems in conversation. Although it is easy to recognize this difficulty in the question and answer conversation paradigm, these children will evidence the same difficulty in
spontaneous conversation. Sometimes adults encourage off target responding
by allowing a child to continue the conversation from whatever topic the child
introduces. For example: "Did you have a good time at the party?" The child
says, "I ate at least three cookies." Even though the question was not answered appropriately, the adult may accept the response and say, "Oh, you ate
cookies at the party." Accepting an inappropriate answer camouflages the rules
of the speech act. More will be said about assessing and treating this problem
in later chapters.

Syntactic Errors

A *syntactic error* is an unconventional ordering of the lexicon (vocabulary).
This problem has been included in semantic and pragmatic disorders because
it's the author's experience that children generally do not have difficulty ordering words unless a basic semantic problem of sequencing of relations exists.
The basic linearity of the English language system is acquired by children at an
early age (Brown, 1973). This linguistic ability remains constant. Most errors
that are referred to as syntactical in nature are really morphological and are related to the child's normal acquisition process or to the significant models in
the environment. The morphological errors, which are structural in nature and
related solely to form, do not affect the function or the content in most inci-
dences. The child's knowledge of the environment is adequate, so that the content and intent of the utterances are well developed and are not misunderstood
by the hearer. An example of a morphological error, from an adult perspective,

has been taken from a five year old who is naturally acquiring English: "Johnny is my bestest friend."

Notice in this example that the word order or syntax has not been altered, but there is an error in the addition of *-est* to a word denoting a superlative (*-est* added to "best" is redundant). Upon questioning, it is obvious that the child's meaning is not redundant. Therefore, the error is of a structural nature, while the meaning or basic semantic understanding remains unchanged.

An error in the ordering of words, which is a syntactic error of the surface structure, usually occurs as a product of a problem in the semantic basis underlying the structure. The following is an example of an utterance with a syntactic transposition: "My house, well, I live in, well, my house, uh, I live in." In this example, the child transposed, or exchanged, the position of the two basic ideas: "my house" and "I live." The child may have intended to say, "I live in my house." Although this utterance would have been grammatically complete, its semantic basis or content is weak unless the context would have demanded a specification of the referent "my house" versus "your house" or "somebody else's house."

Examination of syntactical confusion has led to the temporary conclusion that children who make these errors are experiencing difficulty with the sequencing of referential meaning as the referents relate to a conventional set of suitable topics. Once the child's utterance is put into a grammatical order, the meaning is often not as intended. This indicates a more basic semantic disorder associated with referent choice or meaning. For example, consider the child who says, "The baseball, uh, threw the base." The utterance is then put into grammatical order: "The boy threw the baseball (to the base)." This grammatical utterance is then put into context and it doesn't fit because the context shows the pitcher throwing the ball to the hitter. Of course, the pitcher could be the boy and homeplate could be the base. But when the child is asked to explain the action, he says that the "base" in the original utterance referred to first base, not homeplate. The child's surface order apparently was a product of the underlying semantic confusions.

Syntactic errors almost always are associated with other specific semantic errors indicative of a more general language disorder.

Semantic Word Errors

Selecting an inappropriate word appears to be closely associated with the level of vocabulary development. Chapter 1 described a theoretical position suggesting that vocabulary acquisition is gradual and directly dependent upon the child's level of cognitive knowledge. Based on this literature and the literature on comprehension, production, and imitation, a child may not use a word in all possible adult ways until the child is at an advanced cognitive level. Of course the child may use a word in an adultlike manner on one specific occasion or even on several occasions. But in any given situation, the child may not be able to use a particular word in an adultlike manner.

When the child's process of vocabulary acquisition is distorted or interrupted, the likelihood of misusing a word increases. The child finds it harder and harder to use the lexicon as acquired knowledge outstrips his or her ability to process and associate actions, objects, and/or events with the words. There are several lexical areas of conceptual development that appear to be most affected: space (for example, words denoting position such as "up" or "down"), time (for example, words indicating "before" and "next"), dimensional qualities (for example, opposites of size or shape such as "big" or "little"), other attribute qualifiers (for example, polars of adjectives such as "hot" and "cold"), and quantifiers (for example, words indicating amount such as "more" or "another").

The reader will recall that Chapter 1 presented a basic theoretical position to explain the acquisition of these concepts: namely, that the referential lexicon in a child's language closely represents the acquired level of conceptual knowledge. Therefore a semantic word error represents a disorder in the acquisition of conceptual knowledge. This problem is not a result of the child's lack of experience and should not be confused with the inability to use a word because knowledge of the word does not exist in the child's repertoire. The semantic word error is a product of a child's inability to organize the perceptual and functional attributes into a pattern that constitutes the word.

For example, a child, in order to use the preposition "in" must understand some of the semantic relationships between objects and the spatial concept denoted by the word "in." During a spontaneous language sample, a precocious six-year-old male said, "The chicken is in the dirt." When the planted vegetables were pointed out to the child, he corrected himself and said, "The chicken is on the garden." Although this child was experiencing difficulty choosing the appropriate "in" or "on" preposition, in several other situations the same child chose the correct preposition.

The problem for this child is not vocabulary but semantic relationships. What is the relationship between the chicken and the garden? Or what is the relationship between the garden and the dirt? If a garden is a flat space, then the chicken should be "on" the garden; but if the garden has depth from the plants, fence, and so forth, then the chicken is "in" the garden. Adult usage would usually be "in" since gardens are considered areas and not flat surfaces. As soon as the adult usage is given, however, there will be some reader who will support the boy's usage. This preference appears to be geographically or possibly socioculturally related. In the same way, some people would build "tall" buildings and some people would build "high" buildings (Fleming,

1978). The use of many spatio-temporal and dimensional concepts is regulated by societal conventions.

Another child who experienced difficulty with spatio-temporal terms often perplexed his parents and teachers with behavior that was sometimes interpreted as "acting out." When the child's mother asked him to go get "on" his clothes, he stood on the clothes; a very literal translation of the mother's statement indicating that the child had acquired some knowledge about "in" but did not have enough information for this situation. This same seven-year-old male believed that the building moved while the elevator remained stationary. When asked to find a seat, he wiggled behind some chairs and stood at attention even though the rest of the people in the room were sitting. When a picture of a plane landing was placed on the desktop in front of him, he said that the plane was taking off. If the same picture was placed above his head, he said the plane was flying; if the picture was tilted at eye level, he thought the plane was landing. This child was at age level for all measures of articulation and language, vocabulary comprehension, syntax, and morphology. But all of the perceptual and functional attributes that distinguish the relationships among actions, objects, and events were confusing to this child whose only referent for distinction was his body. He was not able to use the spatial or temporal points of reference provided by the environment.

The child who is having difficulty acquiring the basic semantic relationships—particularly for the spatio-temporal terms, qualifiers, and quantifiers—is often misdiagnosed and/or misunderstood. This child usually acquires the basic agent, action, object relationships, but as the dative, locative and other more complex linguistic semantic relations are developing, the child becomes confused—as often evidenced by a serious personality, raised eyebrows, a forehead furrow, and overt behavior that sometimes seems inappropriate. Relatives, friends, and teachers describe the child as "sounding funny" and later say the child is having academic difficulties.

The child with semantic word errors usually has difficulty with the aforementioned concepts, and these word errors are symptoms of an overall problem that eventually affects the child's syntax and morphology. As the child tries to express how the environment is organized, entire phrases may become entangled. For example: "Sometimes I ride my bike, uh, um, my bike and I ride the bus." "Do you take your bike with you on the bus?" "No, I drive, 'er, ride the bus, you see, and then I ride the bike." Although there are no temporal words in this child's utterances (as will be described in the diagnostic section), this child's sequencing of the phrases indicates a temporal problem, a general language disorder that results in problems with the syntactical relationships.

Progressing through academic stages, the child with this type of semantic difficulty evidences more trouble with language production. Academic deficiencies may show up, particularly in reading and in quantity tasks related to mathematics. This child often develops a visual or sight vocabulary and does not have difficulty with rote math skills that do not require an auditory processing. This child may acquire most knowledge from visual, tactile, kinesthetic, and olfactory experiences. But, to have a complex oral/aural linguistic system, the child must have an auditory system that can use the visual or auditory information.

The children who evidence semantic word errors are often identified as learning disabled and receive special academic services and resource assistance for academic skills. Chapter 4 deals with language remediation approaches found to be effective with this population.

Other children will also evidence the same deficiencies in use of these conceptual terms. Children who are mentally retarded not only develop language at a slower rate than other children (e.g., Karlin, 1952; Kahn, 1975; Lackner, 1968; Lenneberg, Nichols, & Rosenberger, 1969; Miller & Yoder, 1974; and Morehead & Ingram, 1973), but also show disorders in the semantic area of development (Bartel, Bryan, & Keehn, 1973; Schauer, 1978; Semmel, Barritt, & Bennett, 1970). Although the ability to use structure and form is a skill easily learned and trained (e.g., Gray & Ryan, 1973; Kent, 1974; Marshall & Hegrenes, 1970), until recently minimal effort has been aimed at semantic development (McLean & Snyder-McLean, 1978). Those programs that have encouraged early identification and intervention, beginning with the semantic/cognitive language level, have had great success at raising the child's initial academic performance (Hayden, 1979). The author has observed that the longer the mentally retarded child develops syntax and morphology without concentrated effort on the semantic development, the greater the likelihood there will be specific semantic disorders. The literature which compares normal development with that of the mentally retarded child indicates that the conceptual areas of development are greatly affected. Consequently, the semantic word errors (space, time, quantity, and quality) are numerous in these children's language.

Emotionally disturbed children will make semantic word errors that are not so much specific conceptual errors but are more closely related to an inability to express the child's intent. For example, a child might say, "My bird died this morning." The adult might respond, "Your bird died last year." This child's confusion of time is not related to a semantic word error problem that involves inappropriate usage of temporal terms, but is related to the child's psychoeducational needs. The child's real intent was probably not to tell the adult about his bird but to get the adult's attention or perhaps to ask for help with an academic task. When the adult examines the context, there is usually an anxiety-provoking antecedent(s) that encourages this off topic and temporally out of sequence utterance.

There are also some children who make semantic word errors associated with categorical perceptual or functional attributes. Some categories include sizes, shapes, colors, textures, sounds, and purposes. The child perceives relationships in terms of these categories, and this results in unusual usage of some vocabulary terms. A seven-year-old female described the following:

> "A snowman is two circles, like this." (The child drew imaginary circles with her finger.) "Um, an umbrella is a round thing like this." (Again she drew with her finger.) "You use it in the rain. A lamp is a square thing and a circle on top. A hat is two circles like this." (Again she drew a hat composed of two circles, one smaller circle on top of the larger circle.)

This child had a general language disorder with specific language problems, including an obsession for shapes. It was interesting to note that her school report card indicated that she was above the rest of the children in her classroom in matching shapes. Her obsession for shapes explained semantic word errors such as: "What did you have for breakfast?" "I had two circles like this with syrup and butter."

Some children who show severe semantic word errors coupled with syntactic/semantic problems appear to have a fluency problem. For example, consider the adolescent male who functioned at a moderately retarded level in academic situations and was diagnosed as having a severe stuttering problem. Fluency therapy was not effective. The client moved and was rediagnosed at another clinic as having a severe language disorder. The blocks were directly related to an inability to sequence referents. Because this problem was compounded by difficulties with acquiring referential meaning (which by definition is a product of the environment), the client was most dysfluent. Secondary characteristics associated with stuttering were also present. A direct language patterning program (see Chapter 7) with emphasis on acquiring the perceptual and functional semantic attributes of lexicon was quite effective at reducing the client's stuttering behavior. From the adolescent's point of view, it is highly stressful to understand that it's time to speak and not have the right symbols to express one's ideas or intentions.

From the previous examples, it's evident that semantic word errors may be manifested in a variety of forms that all have the same result—an interruption in the flow of ideas. The remediation process is basically the same for the various diagnoses since the underlying difficulty remains constant.

Word-Finding Problems

The literature is replete with descriptions of *anomia* and other word-finding problems associated with trauma or insult in adults and children (e.g., Johnson & Myklebust, 1967; Sarno, 1972; Schuell, Jenkins, & Jimenez-Pabon, 1964). This section will not restate or evaluate the available literature, but will summarize for the clinician the basic distinction between a child with a recall problem versus a child who is unable to use a word because of semantic difficulties. The difference between these two problems will determine the therapeutic method and the effectiveness of the remediation.

If there is a problem recalling a word, the child usually exhibits these linguistic characteristics. The child will describe perceptual and functional attributes, but may not be able to name the action, object, and/or event. For example, "It's, uh, soft, white, and Mom uses it to, uh, to clean the baby." "What's it called?" "I can't remember." An older child may be able to categorize the unnamed item, as well as name other items in the category. For example, "Well, it's a vegetable and it's like potatoes, carrots, onions. They all grow underground." "What's it called?" "I can't remember." (Beets) Action words are less problematic than those words depicting objects and events, since similar action words can be substituted without greatly altering the connotative meaning. For example, "Well he, uh, just hurried right along." ("Ran" was the word the child couldn't remember.) Substitutions make the inability less noticeable to the hearers. Conceptual knowledge is not deficient for the child's cognitive or academic level, unless the word retrieval problem is secondary to more extensive difficulties.

There is another kind of child who appears to have word-finding difficulties but is really struggling with sequencing of the basic semantic relations. The linguistic characteristics of this child include semantic word error problems often coupled with apparent disorganization. The speech pattern is often interrupted so that the child's message becomes dysfluent, but the language problems are creating the disorganized pattern.

There is a major difference between the child with recall word-finding problems and the child with a semantic disorder manifested in word-finding problems: The child with recall problems knows what needs to be said and can't say the idea, whereas the child with the semantic language disorder doesn't really know what to say. Diagnostically the symptoms are different. The child with recall problems can't name but may have adequate conceptual knowledge and may be able to categorize noun vocabulary. Chapter 4 discusses further diagnostic distinctions between these two types of children.

Neologisms

Neologisms (newly created words), like word-finding difficulties, have been discussed in the literature particularly in regard to aphasic and brain damaged clients (DeRenzi, Pieczuro, & Vignolo, 1972; Geschwind, 1972; Weinstein et al., 1972). Neologisms may be created in three basic ways: structural, semantic, and phonological.

The first type, created from structural changes, occurs when syllables are scrambled. For example, "helicopter" is consistently produced as "copihelter." A semantic neologism occurs when the speaker uses a word that has a similar connotative meaning such as "pull-ons" for "boots." Similar sound exchanges create phonological neologisms, as when "bread" is changed to "brad." The use of the neologism is usually consistent, unless the child's feedback system fluctuates so that on some days the child can unscramble or decode phonological or structural similarities and differences. The semantic neologism is much more consistent than the other two types and is easier to change in therapy.

A child who appears to be using a structural neologism such as "copihelter" will usually exhibit other difficulties in organizing semantic relations. As mentioned previously, as the linguistic expression of these semantic relations becomes more difficult, the general language disorder becomes more obvious. Semantic neologisms, or the creation of substitute words, are often part of a child's problem in understanding the perceptual and functional attributes of words. This may be due to a visual acuity and/or visual motor problem or a distorted perspective of reality as might be found with emotionally disturbed children. Children who have difficulty acquiring perceptual and functional attributes may emphasize one feature of an object, action, and/or event over other features. For example, one child insisted on a "plane" being a "fly" throughout a lengthy story because the picture of the plane showed two wings. This child's rigidity illustrates how these children often interpret things literally because their attention is focused on one feature. In another example of literality, consider the child who insisted that a certain part of town was called "junior police streets," an excellent semantic neologism, because the child was part of the junior police who patrolled those streets. The adults listening to the child's story could not understand the condensation of meaning into the phrase "junior police streets," and would say that the child was not making sense. Thus the child's communicative attempt was not effective.

Phonological neologisms occur quite frequently with auditory misperceptions. An example of intentional phonological neologism can be found on television in beer commercials that depict a person using odd combinations of syllables (spoonerisms) that closely resemble the correct auditory production. The author has found that phonological neologisms are not so much an indicator of an extensive language problem as are the structural and semantic neologisms.

Topical or Referential Identification Problems

As a hearer scans a speaker's message, the salient features of the message are used to maintain the topic. Saliency depends on the listener's previous experiences as well as on the current setting and context. Since the normal speaker/hearer setting requires a conventional form of communication to be effective, the hearer must be able to identify the speaker's referent or the contextual referents in order to maintain the conversation. Because some children have difficulty selecting the appropriate referent, their answers to questions or their attempts to continue the topic of conversation are ineffective.

Problems with inappropriate topical or referential identification are most significant with respect to asking and answering questions. The child's difficulty here is directly related to the complexity of the question or the required answer. To answer a question, the child must be able to recognize the referent of the speaker's utterance and then have the knowledge and linguistic skills necessary for answering. An example of inappropriate topic identification follows:

> "Sally, did you put your homework on my desk?"
> "Ms. Smith, my desk is clean."
> "Good, did you put your homework on *my* desk?"
> "Here is my homework."
> "What did I ask about your homework?"
> "Put it on my desk?"
> "No." I said, "Did you put your homework on *my* desk?"
> "Oh!"

The child is listening to various segments of the teacher's utterances but is unable to identify the topic (where the homework is located) and, in this case, is unable to determine the comment about the topic.

This semantic error may appear to overlap with off target responding as previously described. However, there is one basic difference between the two semantic disorders: In off target responding the child is apparently satisfied with the utterance, although it may not even be related to the situation or to the previous utterances. In poor topic or referent identification the response is directly related to the situation and/or the previous utterances, but the child usually is not satisfied. This lack of satisfaction is seen in the child's searching for the salient information.

The longer the speaker's utterances and the greater the semantic load being conveyed, the more complex is the cognitive information needed to respond, and the greater the likelihood of showing topical identification problems. For example, in the specific question, "What are you eating?" it is easier for a child to identify the referent than in the question, "What's happening in the story?" which requires the child to make some inferences and possibly come to some conclusions.

Topic Closure Difficulties

This problem is often the most baffling for those individuals desperately trying to improve language in one child and at the same time finding it impossible to communicate effectively with a child who never stops talking. Children who have a problem with topic closure cannot determine the boundaries of their utterances in terms of ideas or topics. Consequently, they continue to talk.

Boundaries are arbitrary, rather than grammatical, divisions around ideas or semantic bits of information that a speaker wishes to convey to a hearer. *Pauses* and other prosodic devices are used to linguistically mark the divisions between the boundaries. The child who has difficulty with determining the beginnings and ends of bits of information intended to affect some change in the hearer will continue to rephrase, reword, or reiterate the message until either an environmental or inner stop is employed. This type of excessive verbalization is often as serious, and as frustrating to a hearer as another child's lack of language skills. The author's experience with these children suggests that children without boundary limitation need structure in organizing the content of their messages.

Consider the following segment of conversation taken from an eleven-year-old female described by the teacher as "motor mouth."

> "Well, hello. I said, hello. How are you today? What are we going to do? Are we going to make pictures in art? Are we going to make art pictures? (The teacher asks her if she wants to make art pictures.) Well, I don't know. I don't know if I want to do art today. My fingers are sore. See, my fingers are sore. I'm not sure if I want to do art. What are we going to do today? Do we have to make pictures in art? I really don't know if I can make a picture in art—etc., etc., etc."

Tangentiality

If a child makes an association with a spoken or contextual referent prior to speaking, the product is a *tangential utterance*. Normal speakers often produce tangential utterances that sometimes necessitate a quick explanation or a polite excuse for deviating from the present subject. An example of an association or tangential utterance is taken from a six-year-old male:

> "John, pick up the red book."
> John picks up the red truck and says, "Truck!"

A young child will substitute other members of a word class that syntactically are likely to precede or follow the associated word, a syntagmatic association. In this instance the adjective "red" is followed by a noun, either "book" or another noun "truck." The association between "book" and "truck" is "red," an adjective or qualifier that could precede either noun.

An older child will make a *paradigmatic association*, an association with another member of the same word class. To the question, "John, pick up the red book," the older child might respond, "I don't have a yellow one." Another example might go as follows:

"John, did you have a banana for lunch?"
John replies, "Yes, apples."

John may or may not have had apples; the referent is unclear. Although associations result in tangential utterances, those associations that are similar to the topic but not quite the same are difficult to recognize. If the associations can be identified, then the specific problem can be directly considered in therapy.

Echolalia

One of the most perplexing disorders of speech and language is *echolalia*, or the listener's restatement of a speaker's previously uttered words, phrases, paragraphs, etc. The literature regarding the brain damaged child and the emotionally disturbed child has discussed this phenomenon from several theoretical and remediational perspectives (e.g., Bartak & Rutter, 1973; Cunningham & Dixon, 1961; Graziano, 1971; Hartung, 1970; Hewett, 1965; Jensen & Womack, 1967; Kanner, 1942; Kanner, 1944; Oppenheim, 1974; Ricks & Wing, 1975; Risley & Wolf, 1967; Ritvo, 1976; Schell, Stark, & Giddan, 1967; Sloane & MacAulay, 1968; Yule & Berger, 1975). The purpose of dealing with echolalia in this chapter on semantic and pragmatic disorders is to highlight the involved language disorders as well as illustrate the differences between the grammatical level of echolalia (linguistic performance) and the child's semantic level of linguistic competence.

There has been much written about the imitation/competence/performance issue as it relates to the comprehension of the speaker and hearer, but the discussion has been inconclusive. It should be stressed that the elicited and direct imitation discussed in the literature is significantly different from a child's echolalic production. The echolalic utterance usually lacks prosodic features that would characterize the same utterance as meaningful. Furthermore, the echolalic utterance is quite frequently more grammatically complete than is the speaker's comprehension of the utterance. This does not necessarily contradict the literature indicating that linguistic competence and performance are at least parallel. The child is obviously capable of producing the linguistic string, so production and the competence to produce are the same; but the comprehension is being challenged in the case of echoed utterances. The level of comprehension appears to be lower than the grammatical level represented by the echoed utterances.

During a diagnostic evaluation, the diagnostician may be able to converse with the echolalic child on a very simple non-echoed linguistic level. But once the grammatical demands of the clinician's utterances challenge the child, the echolalia increases. It appears that the echolalic utterances lack the advanced semantic meaning implied by the echoed structural or grammatical level. Therefore, it is critical that the clinician be able to determine the spontaneous language level as well as the imitated level. Because echolalic utterances lack the meaning represented by the echoed utterance, this problem will be treated as a semantic language disorder. More specifically, the advanced semantic sequencing according to environmental associations appears to be deviant in echolalia.

Verbal Perseveration

Verbal perseveration refers to the reiteration of a word, phrase, sentence, or idea. Different from echolalia, the utterance or idea that is perseverated begins in a meaningful context and is then perpetuated. The prosodic features are as natural as the original meaningful utterances, and removal of the context or triggering situation alleviates that moment of perseveration. Furthermore, the perseveration occurs at the child's spontaneous linguistic level. The literature on brain damaged children and adults deals with perseveration as a motor or verbal behavior (e.g., Sarno, 1972).

In the following segment, the child rewords, rephrases, and reiterates the same idea, words, and/or phrases regarding an art assignment:

"Ms. Smith, what's the paper for?"
"Johnny, it's for the art lesson."
"Ms. Smith, what's the paper for?"
"It's for the art lesson."
"Ms. Smith, tell me, what's the paper for?"
"Johnny, I already told you."
"Ms. Smith, tell me it's for the art lesson. The paper is for the art lesson."
"Johnny, the paper is for the art lesson."
"Ms. Smith, tell me what the paper is for."
Etc.

In another case, a six-year-old female who was engaged in a pretend tea party when she began to stir in the coffee cup and chat about "coffee, cream, and sugar . . . ." Once the child began the motor routine of stirring paired with the verbalization, she could not be physically or verbally redirected nor could the topic be changed until the clinician took the child into a different room. Verbal and motor perseveration often appear to be paired together.

Phonological Problems

The symptoms of phonological language disorder are not as easy to describe as with the previous semantic problems. Characteristically, the child with this disorder is usually younger than eight or nine and is unintelligible to most hearers. This child is often treated for articulation errors, but closer examination of the child's language reveals frequent syllable omission and inconsistent use of functors. This *phonological disorder* may be approached from several theoretical perspectives including analyzing distinctive features (e.g., McReynolds & Bennett, 1972; Pollack & Rees, 1972), writing the phonological rules for the child (e.g., Ingram, 1974, 1976), or using a multiple phonemic approach (Bradley & McCabe, 1974).

This particular phonological disorder has been included under semantic problems because the errors are morphophonemic in nature; the child has difficulty with more than just sound production, as might be the case with an articulation disorder. This child omits meaningful units such as auxiliary verbs and articles by altering the conventional rules that govern morpheme combinations. It is likely that the child has an individual, but systematic, set of rule formulations. Therefore, a four-year-old child who says, "Da ma daw" may be enrolled in articulation therapy; but this child should have at least said, "Da e ma daw" for "That is my dog," if the problem were purely articulatory or linked to motor production.

The omission of the functors or syllables, particularly at the ends of words that require inflectional morphemes, is a key to the diagnosis and treatment. A few comments regarding treatment will be made in Chapter 7, but it should be clear that most of these children are not assisted by traditional articulation therapy. Language development must be fostered either through peer models and patterns of intervention or through some other direct phonological perspective.

This particular disorder differs from the others mentioned in this chapter in that it is the only disorder that deals directly with the sound and morpheme rule system. But this disorder has more similarities than differences with the other disorders. In terms of the speech act, this child has a problem with the essential rule components or linguistic expression. A child with a phonological problem appears to understand the propositional, sincerity, and preparatory rules, but still has difficulty performing successful speech acts because the hearer can't understand the child and therefore cannot be affected as the child intended.

Summary of Semantic Language Disorders

Whenever a semantic language disorder occurs, there is an effect on language usage. The degree of effect depends directly on the extent or frequency of semantic disruption as well as on the place of breakdown (that is, on the in-

put, output, or processing). In a reasonable sense, if the child is having difficulty receiving and interpreting the semantic relations in the environment, then
the cumulative effect on the child's language will be greater than if the problem
is in communicating an intended message to a hearer. It should be noted that
the majority of observable language disorders have their basis in the interpretation and comprehension of language. Therefore, a semantic language disorder
results in a pragmatic problem.

The semantic deviations described here are unusual linguistic behaviors
which, when present, are indicative of a disordered language system. However,
a child's language doesn't necessarily need to evidence any one or all of these
specific symptoms to be considered disordered. In fact, a child's language may
be disordered when a specific area of linguistic acquisition (phonology, syntax,
morphology, semantics) is no longer following a systematic or sequential pattern of development. Furthermore, whenever a child is no longer pragmatically
appropriate, the language usage problem indicates a disorder in one of the areas
of language—specifically, semantics. There are children who experience some
difficulty in using language skills as intended (shy or reticent children, for example), but the appropriateness of the language usage is satisfactory at most
times and in most situations. Excessive reticence would affect the child's overall functioning and would be a language disorder associated with pragmatics.
These children's difficulties may be traced back to problems in the semantic
rules of the speech act.

DISRUPTION OF THE SPEECH ACT

Children who evidence problems with acquiring the semantic rules of the
speech act are not able to complete a high enough percentage of speech acts to
be judged effective communicators. The essential, preparatory, propositional
content, and/or sincerity rules are violated.

The following hypothetical example uses the speech act rules described in
Chapter 2 to analyze a breakdown in communicating an intended message.
Each of the rules corresponding to the hypothetical context has been delineated,
so the reader may observe the breakdown of communication as a disruption of
speech act rules.

Context: The classroom setting with the teacher and John about ten feet apart
at the beginning of the speech act.

Preparatory Rule: John wants the paper on the teacher's desk. He does not
realize (violation of this rule) that to obtain the paper he must ask the
teacher. (Without an utterance, a speech act is not attempted.)

Propositional Content Rule: Since the preparatory rule has been violated,
John will attempt to physically obtain the paper without an utterance.

Since there is no utterance that specifies the child's intent, the chance that the child's physical behavior will be misunderstood is increased. The use of specific linguistic skills increases the likelihood of understanding the communication in situations in which the conventional mode is aural/oral.

Sincerity Rule: The speech act is not attempted, and it is obvious what John wants.

Essential Rule: John does turn toward the teacher, indicating that he wants the teacher's attention. Then he turns toward the desk, signaling his focus of attention on the desk. But John has failed to get the paper.

In the next example there is an utterance, but there is a breakdown because of violation of the rules.

Context: The classroom and the teacher.

Preparatory Rule: John knows that to receive the paper on the teacher's desk, he must obtain it from the teacher.

Propositional Content Rule: It is obvious to John and to the teacher that he needs to ask for the paper. John says, "Give it, please." Because the utterance does not specify the referent "paper," confusion may result.

Sincerity Rule: The child does want "X," and the teacher recognizes his need.

Essential Rule: The child does get the teacher's attention by looking at her, but he doesn't look at the paper while making the utterance. Since his utterance lacks referential clarity, the teacher is unsure as to what the child wants.

In the last example the child attempted a speech act to get the hearer to do something for him, but the speech act lacked the necessary components to make it a complete or effective form of linguistic communication.

There are an infinite number of ways to perform a speech act and thus an equal number of ways to violate the semantic rules that constitute the speech act. It is not surprising then that there is so much misunderstanding among speakers. The problem with many language disordered children is that although the linguistic form may be taught as a structural skill, pattern, or task, there is a lack of knowledge of the underlying semantic relations for the preparatory rule as well as an inability to organize the environment by referents and their relationships to physical and linguistic behavior. Therefore, any time a semantic disorder occurs, there will be some effect on the pragmatic aspects of language. Similarly, an obvious problem in being an effective communicator has its roots in the semantic rules.

Although the last set of examples were of speech acts, it is important to give some consideration to the concept of the speech event. A speech event as defined (Dore, 1973; Hymes, 1972) in Chapter 2 includes the performance of several speech acts that have a shared topic and an appropriate context. Certain academic skills or more advanced linguistic behavior (such as *discussing*) are dependent upon the ability to perform more than a single speech act. The following is a segment of conversation taken from a child/adult interaction. The segment has been analyzed according to the rules for a speech act so that whether there is a complete speech act or a disruption in communication, it may be highlighted. The child is a three-year-old female who is linguistically advanced.

1. Adult says, "Karen, where shall we sit?"
   (Speech act: request information)
   [Context: trying to decide where to sit for lunch]

2. Adult says, "We better go into the dining room?"
   (Speech act: rule order)
   [Preparatory: each isn't sure what the other knows]
   (Essential components complete)
   [Sincerity: both want to eat lunch]

3. "Oh, I want to eat here." (joking)
   [Context: adult is pretending to get ready to eat in living room]
   (Speech act: denial of present event)
   [Preparatory: child never eats in living room so she does not have that experience]
   [Sincerity: violated by speaker—essential components are recognized as different by the child]

4. "You, silly. You ate like that!" (pointing)
   (Speech act: assertion)
   [Context: same]   [preparatory: same]
   [Sincerity: child wants to tell adult that the adult is silly]
   [Essential components: linguistic portion is incomplete because the referent for "that" is unclear to hearer]

5. Child says, "You hear the teletype?"
   (Speech act: request for information)
   Proposition: "You hear Y?"
                " X — Y?" Yes or no?

[Context: both go sit at the table to eat]
[Preparatory: not sure if the hearer hears the noise]
[Sincerity: all essential elements indicate child does want the information]
[Essential: complete]

6. Adult says, "How does a teletype work, Karen?"
   (Speech act: request for information)
   Proposition: "Teletype works Y?"
   "   X   –   Y   "
   [Context: same]
   [Preparatory: child doesn't know that the adult is checking information]
   [Sincerity is established]
   [Essential: complete]

7. Child says, "The teletype is, uh, comes out."
   (Speech act: statement of information)
   Proposition: Teletype Y
                 X   –Y
   [Context: same]
   [Preparatory: child wants to explain because she doesn't think the hearer knows]
   [Sincerity is established]
   [Essential: incomplete. Child doesn't have the referential knowledge to explain the task]

8. Child then says, "I hear Cinderella!"
   (Speech act: statement of information)
   Proposition: X hears Y
   [Context: same but Cinderella is a record on the stereo in the living room]
   [Preparatory: child isn't sure the adult hears it *and* previous task was too difficult so new topic is needed]
   [Essential: complete]

An analysis of the eight utterances as part of a speech event indicates that there were six speech acts and two attempts. The two incomplete performances were a result of incomplete linguistic information. The child was too young to express referential meaning in these two incomplete performances, so the utterances lacked referential clarity. Even in a normal conversation between an adult and a linguistically advanced child, there are communicative situations that are not perfect. Any child's language may be analyzed in this way to determine its effectiveness or to trace a difficulty in the semantic rule development.

SEVERITY OF LANGUAGE DISORDER

The severity of disorder depends on several factors including local determinants. Many states are adopting severity indices to determine how much disorder must be measured by a standardized instrument to warrant placement in a special services program and to establish how much time the clinician is allowed to work with the client. With regard to the semantic/pragmatic language disorders described there, severity is based on the distinction between delay and disorder as well as on the amount of deviation from a child's normative expectation. But more importantly, the severity should also be determined by the degree of academic and social effects that can only be assessed by a thorough language evaluation (to be discussed in the next chapter). The distinction between delays and disorders is critical to the prognosis as well as to the chosen remediation procedures. The type of approach used to facilitate delayed language should be different from the approach used to remediate the unsystematic and/or nonsequential language acquisition. This book is concerned with semantic and pragmatic disorders; the clinician should realize that the techniques and procedures described here are designed to intervene and remediate and are not aimed at habilitation of normal language acquisition.

SUMMARY

A child who is slower to develop a language system than other children of the same chronological age is considered language delayed since the systematic and sequential properties are maintained. If the delay is persistent, it may result in a language disorder since development of the more advanced semantic skills is interrupted. Language disorders also occur as a product of underlying changes, interruptions, and deviations in the development of semantics. Several specific symptoms or language disorders do emerge as distinct problems requiring special remediation programs. Chapter 4 discusses the identification of these specific language disorders.

Questions

1. Why does this chapter place so much importance on semantic development?
2. What is the relationship between the specific semantic problems and a general inability to be pragmatically skillful?
3. What is the clinical significance of understanding the semantic problems?
4. What, if any, advantage is there in describing language problems without specific descriptions based on diagnoses such as mental retardation?
5. Which semantic problems overlap with each other?

REFERENCES

Bartak, L., & Rutter, M. Special educational treatment of autistic children: A comparative study. *Journal of Child Psychology and Psychiatry,* 1973, *14,* 161-179.

Bartel, N. R., Bryan, D., & Keehn, S. Language comprehension in the moderately retarded child. *Exceptional Child,* 1973, *39,* 375-382.

Bradley, D. P., & McCabe, R. B. Systematic multiple-phonemic approach to articulation therapy. *Acta Symbolica,* 1974, *6* (1), 2-17.

Brown, R. *A first language: The early stages.* Cambridge, Mass.: Harvard University Press, 1973.

Cunningham, M. A., & Dixon, C. A. A study of the language of an autistic child. *Journal of Child Psychology and Psychiatry,* 1961, *2,* 193-202.

DeRenzi, E., Pieczuro, A., Vignolo, L. A. Oral apraxia and aphasia. In M. T. Sarno (Ed.), *Aphasia: Selected readings.* Englewood Cliffs, New Jersey: Prentice-Hall, 1972.

Dore, J. The development of speech acts. (Doctoral dissertation, City University of New York, 1973). *Dissertation Abstracts International,* 1973, *34* (University Microfilms No. 73-14, 374).

Fleming, K. A. Preschool children's performances on spatial locative *high* tasks. An unpublished manuscript, Washington State University, 1978.

Geschwind, N. The varieties of naming errors. In M. T. Sarno (Ed.), *Aphasia: Selected readings.* Englewood Cliffs, New Jersey: Prentice-Hall, 1972.

Gray, B. B., & Ryan, B. P. *A language program for the non-language child.* Champaign, Il.: Research Press, 1973.

Graziano, A. (Ed.). *Behavior therapy with children.* Chicago, Il.: Aldine, 1971.

Hartung, J. A., Jr. A review of procedures to increase verbal imitation skills and functional speech in autistic children. *Journal of Speech and Hearing Disorders,* 1970, *35,* 203-216.

Hayden, A. H. Implications of infant intervention research. *Allied Health and Behavioral Sciences,* 1979, *1* (4).

Hewett, F. M. Teaching speech to an autistic child through operant conditioning. *American Journal of Orthopsychiatry,* 1965, *34,* 927-936.

Hymes, D. Models of the interaction of language and social life. In J. Gumperz & D. Hymes (Eds.), *Directions in sociolinguistics.* New York: Holt, Rinehart, & Winston, 1972.

Ingram, D. Phonological rules in young children. *Journal of Child Language,* 1974, *1,* 49-64.

Ingram, D. *Phonological disability in children.* New York: Elsevier North Holland, 1976.

Jensen, G. P., & Womack, M. G. Operant conditioning techniques applied in the treatment of an autistic child. *American Journal of Orthopsychiatry,* 1967, *37,* 30-35.

Johnson, D. L., & Myklebust, H. R. *Learning disabilities: Educational principles and practices.* New York: Grune and Stratton, 1967.

Kahn, J. Relationship of Piaget's sensorimotor period to language acquisition of profoundly retarded children. *American Journal of Mental Deficiency,* 1975, *79,* 640-644.

Kanner, L. Autistic disturbances of affective contact. *The Nervous Child,* 1942, *2,* 217-251.

Kanner, L. Early infantile autism. *Journal of Pediatrics,* 1944, *25,* 211-217.

Karlin, I. W. Speech and language problems of mentally deficient children. *Journal of Speech and Hearing Disorders,* 1952, *17,* 286-294.

Kent, L. R. *Language acquisition program for the severely retarded.* Champaign, Ill.: Research Press, 1974.

Lackner, J. R. A developmental study of language behavior in retarded children. *Neuropsychologia,* 1968, *6,* 301-320.

Lenneberg, E. H., Nichols, I. A., & Rosenberger, E. F. Premature stages in language development in monogolism. In D. M. Rioch & E. A. Weinstein (Eds.), *Disorders of communication.* New York: Hafner Publishing Co., 1969.

Marshall, N., & Hegrenes, T. Programmed communication therapy for autistic mentally retarded children. *Journal of Speech and Hearing Disorders,* 1970, *35,* 70-83.

McLean, J. & Snyder-McLean, L. *A transactional approach to early language training.* Columbus, Ohio: Charles E. Merrill, 1978.

McReynolds, L. V., & Bennett, S. Distinctive feature generalization in articulation training. *Journal of Speech and Hearing Disorders,* 1972, *37,* 462-471.

Miller, J. F., & Yoder, D. E. An ontogenetic language teaching strategy for retarded children. In R. L. Schiefelbusch & L. L. Lloyd (Eds.). *Language perspectives, acquisition, and retardation.* Baltimore, Md.: University Park Press, 1974.

Morehead, D. M., & Ingram, D. The development of base syntax in normal and linguistically deviant children. *Journal of Speech and Hearing Research,* 1973, *16,* 330-352.

Oppenheim, R. C. *Effective teaching methods for autistic children.* Springfield, Ill.: Charles C. Thomas, 1974.

Pollack, E., & Rees, N. S. Disorders of articulation: Some clinical applications of distinctive feature theory. *Journal of Speech and Hearing Disorders,* 1972, *37,* 447-451.

Ricks, D. M., & Wing, L. Language, communication, and the use of symbols in normal and autistic children. *Journal of Autism and Childhood Schizophrenia,* 1975, *5* (3), 191-221.

Risley, T., & Wolf, M. Establishing functional speech in echolalic children. *Behavior Research and Therapy,* 1967, *5,* 73-88.

Ritvo, E. R. (Ed.). *Autism.* New York: Spectrum Publications, 1976.

Sarno, M. T. (Ed.). *Aphasia: Selected readings.* Englewood Cliffs, New Jersey: Prentice-Hall, 1972.

Schauer, M. *Qualitative analyses of retarded vs. normal children's language samples.* Unpublished master's project, Washington State University, 1978.

Schell, R. E., Stark, J., & Giddan, J. J. Development of language behavior in an autistic child. *Journal of Speech and Hearing Disorders,* 1967, *32,* 51-64.

Schuell, H., Jenkins, J. J., & Jimenez-Pabon, E. (Eds.). *Aphasia in Adults.* New York: Harper & Row, 1964.

Semmel, M. I., Barritte, L. S., & Bennett, S. W. Performance of EMR and nonretarded children on a modified close task. *American Journal of Mental Deficiency,* 1970, *74,* 681-688.

Sloane, H. W., & MacAulay, B. D. *Operant procedures in remedial speech and language training.* Boston: Houghton Mifflin, Co., 1968.

Weinstein, E. A., Lyerly, O. G., Cole, M., & Ozer, M. N. Meaning in jargon aphasia. In M. T. Sarno (Ed.). *Aphasia: Selected readings*. Englewood Cliffs, New Jersey: Prentice-Hall, 1972.

Yule, W., & Berger, M. Communication, language, and behavior modification. In C. C. Kiernan & F. P. Woodford (Eds.). *Behavior modification and the severely retarded*. New York: Elsevier, 1975.

CHAPTER OBJECTIVES

- list the questions used to explain the qualitative properties of a child's language.

- explain each of the questions used to qualitatively analyze the language sample.

- describe the relationship between the language sample and standardized tests.

- list and describe the variables affecting a child's pragmatic language.

- explain the basic variables of obtaining a language sample.

- qualitatively analyze a child's language sample.

- explain the relationship between the qualitative and quantitative analysis of a language sample.

- describe the behavioral observations that indicate that a child has a pragmatic language disorder.

- administer the Behavioral Inventory of Speech Act Performances (BISAP).

- explain the basic difference between criterion referenced and norm referenced tests.

Chapter 4

Assessment and Identification Procedures for Semantic and Pragmatic Language Disorders

A child's linguistic thumbprint
is an illumination of the mind.

This chapter presents methods for qualitatively analyzing language samples, followed by procedures for comparing and substantiating the identification of specific language disorders through standardized tests and behavioral observations. This chapter has been divided into two main sections: (1) language sample analyses; and (2) criterion referenced testing. The section on language sample analyses includes both quantitative and qualitative processes of determining language problems. The section on criterion referenced measures describes an approach to formal assessment of pragmatic and semantic language abilities.

LANGUAGE SAMPLE ANALYSES

Quantitative Measures

There are currently many ways of quantitatively analyzing the structure of language from a language sample. The most commonly used methods include determining the following: Mean Length of Utterance (MLU); Mean Length of Response (MLR), and other associated structural indices; and the Developmental Sentence Score (DSS). These measures are presented in this chapter to give the reader a chance to compare structural and quantitative methods to descriptive methods in order to appreciate the scope and purpose of doing a qualitative analysis. When a clinician is able to distinguish between the types of information obtained from the present quantitative and qualitative methods, then an appropriate assessment of semantics is likely to occur.

The Mean Length of Utterance (for explanation of MLU, see Brown, 1973) is usually calculated as the total number of morphemes in a given number of consecutive utterances divided by the number of utterances. This type of analysis is sensitive to the child's acquisition of morphemes, such as the *s* that denotes plurals when added to a regular noun. The acquisition of meaningful suffixes and the acquisition of the functors (such as *a, the, on,* etc.) is particularly sensitive to this measure.

During the normal language acquisition process, most children pass through a modulation of meaning period around 18 to 40 months of age. This acquisition period is best for using the MLU as a sensitive quantitative measure since it assesses morphological development. Once the child's language acquisition increases beyond this level (MLU = 3.5 to 4.0), the sensitivity decreases and the usefulness of the MLU as a measure of growth or language acquisition decreases. For example, a child might say, "The dog/s jump/ed big," which receives a morpheme count of six. If morphemes were not counted, the child would not receive credit for the plural or for the past tense. However, an adult might say, "Put him on the previous payroll," which would also receive a count of six morphemes. In fact, in true adult conversation, the chance of getting an average (MLU) that is much greater than six is most unlikely. Only if the speaker were lecturing, describing something, or reporting a story would this average be greater. Therefore, the effectiveness of the MLU as a sensitive quantitative measure plateaus after the period characterized by the modulation of meaning through morpheme acquisition.

The mean length of response (MLR) was part of the pioneer language analysis work accomplished by McCarthy and Templin (Johnson, Darley, & Spriestersbach, 1963). The MLR is one of several structural analyses based on the theoretical premise that the child's language abilities increase as the length and structural complexity of the utterance increases (Longhurst, 1974). The MLR is calculated by dividing the total number of words by the total number of utterances in the sample. This type of analysis is a rough index of structural change in language development. Since the child's semantic development is not directly considered, this index is not sensitive to linguistic refinement as the child acquires morphological inflections and more complex forms. Some of the other structural methods reported by Johnson et al. included the structural complexity scores (SCS), the number of different words used in the sample (NDW), and the mean of the mean of the five longest responses. It's beyond the scope of this text to explain these measures except to say that these measures are based on "increases in structural complexity being better" and that they lack sensitivity to semantic influences. (For an in-depth explanation, see Johnson et al., 1963.)

The Developmental Sentence Scoring (DSS) is a process of language sample analysis developed by Laure Lee (1974). The DSS is a quantitative measure of the child's increasing structural complexity, especially as it relates to the development of verb forms. Although the score is quantitative, this DSS method can provide some qualitative data by determining the variety, frequency, and various types of constructions or forms used in each of these adult categorizations: indefinite pronouns or noun modifiers, personal pronouns, main verbs, secondary verbs, negatives, conjunctions, interrogative reversals, wh- questions.

Since a child's verb complexity continues to develop for a longer period of overall language development than other word class constructions, the DSS may be used as a quantitative assessment for older children who are beyond the range of the MLU. Lee provides percentiles for a small group of normative data up to age seven plus. Since a child's basic structural linguistic system should be fairly complete by this age, this measure is quite practical for children with language delays. The development of systematic and sequential rules in the language delayed child may be compared to Lee's normative data, providing that the child fits the population profile.

The previously cited measures are the most common quantitative methods used to determine a child's level of linguistic structural development of morphemes, words, sentences, word classes, and so forth. Other less common quantitative sampling methods include: Tyack's sampling procedures (1973, 1974); Hannah's Linguistic Analysis (1974); the sampling portion of Mac-Donald and Nikols' Environmental Language Inventory (1974); and Crystal's (Crystal, Fletcher, & Garman, 1976) LARSP grammatical analysis (1979), which includes a morphological component that may prove useful in semantic analysis.

There are several common characteristics among the quantitative methods presently available:

1. The methods are aimed at determining the complexity of the structures, with the major underlying premise being that the more "units" the child puts together, the better the child's language. From a semantic-pragmatic viewpoint, once a child is capable of consistently and for a variety of purposes performing a speech act, then the child is communicatively competent and structural development will follow. In other words, the child with truly functional language has the skills to improve complexity.

2. The listed linguistic measures are quantitative unless the clinician is able to interpret the results well enough to do a qualitative analysis of the measured units. In some methods, the total procedure does include an interpretation of the units or constructions used. This structural approach is adequate for syntax and morphological development, but if the child's problem rests in the semantic and pragmatic areas, then the obtained numbers and grammatical analyses do not explain the disorders.

3. For most measures that analyze the forms of structures, the sensitivity implies the development of increasingly more difficult morphological and syntactic skills. Therefore, the best children to evaluate by these quantitative structural methods are those who are developing language in a systematic and primarily sequential order. This means that these methods, supplemented by some other measures that assess academic skills and comprehension and production of language as compared to a normative group of data, are effective evaluation instruments for the delayed language user. Unfortunately, by the time the professional intervenes, most of the children needing special language facilitation are not simply language delayed but language disordered. *When the sequential and/or systematic order of language development is disrupted, the child's acquisition of structures and forms generally will not progress in a normal and organized manner.* Quantitative analyses of language samples may point to the fact that the child has a language problem, but these measures cannot determine what the problems are. This is when the need for qualitative language analysis becomes apparent.

Qualitative Measures

Guidelines for Obtaining Language Samples

There are some basic techniques that should be used if a language sample is to be representative and spontaneous. A representative sample should consist of enough utterances (usually 50, but with low verbal output this may be reduced to 25) that are the best examples of what the child is competent of producing. Spontaneous utterances should not be direct imitations or recognized as indirect imitations. A representative and spontaneous sample may be obtained by using the appropriate materials, context, and adult utterances.

Since the context does influence the content of the child's utterances (Holland, 1975), the sampling materials should be selected to generate a variety of concepts and ideas. The materials should be at the child's level of interaction and cognitive ability. For a child under three years of age (assuming the cognitive level of functioning matches the chronological age), the materials should consist of environmental objects, play toys, and daily activities. Children between the ages of three and seven will limit their play to role playing activities, so many of their utterances are indirect or direct imitations of parents. Often their play conditions produce conversation that, although spontaneous, is not representative. So for a child between three and seven, the materials should consist of play and experience types of pictures. The experience pictures are particularly useful for five- to seven-year-old children. Above seven years of age, the child's stories generated by pictures or conversation about experiences such as hobbies, after-school activities, or school routines are appropriate. Again, these ages are not just chronological indices but are also related to language level.

The context for language sampling should be natural and conducive to spontaneity. The most spontaneous conversations are regulated by the adult speaker's utterances. The adult's tone or mood in talking to the child presets the conditions of the context. From a speech act perspective, the adult establishes the preparatory and, to a significant extent, the propositional content rules from the context conditions.

The adult's or sampler's utterances should be nondirective, appropriately interesting, and responsive to the child. Nondirective utterances include the following: statements or declaratives (rather than interrogatives or questions); short comments about the child's utterances (rather than expatiations about the topic); and parallel play types of utterances. These nondirective utterances should indicate that the adult is interested in *what* the *child* is saying, not how the child is saying it. For example, a "wow" from the adult will keep the child talking more freely than will a response like, "I saw a really great hippopotamus at the Brooklyn Zoo in New York last summer." The interjection, "wow," is a response to the child's talking that shows interest in what the child says. The longer, more complex utterance concentrates on the adult's ideas and not on the child's ideas. The adult should follow the child's verbal lead as much as possible. This pattern of responding may be facilitated by using a few minutes to set the context.

When play materials are available, the play can be directed by comments such as "Here comes Bert. He's a friend of Cookie Monster." Comments like these are preferable to questions like "Do you know who these puppets are?" The comment sets the tone for an equal authoritarian or at least a play relationship between the adult and the child. The question places adult authoritarian stress on the child. With pictures or stories, the adult can set the conditions with an initial model plus directions. For example: "We're going to talk about some pictures. I'll tell a story about this first picture, and then you tell me a story about each of these." The adult provides a complete but linguistically simple story about the first picture. The child now has a model for the task. Most children are reticent to verbalize with an adult, particularly if the home environment suggests that children should be seen and not heard.

If a child's verbal output under sampling conditions is restricted—that is, if the child does not use a variety of forms, structures, functions, and/or speech acts without showing an obvious semantic problem—then the child may need to be tested under different conditions. The sampler may want to go listen to the child in a more natural setting in which the child can interact freely with peers. Another approach is to ask the child to come to the sampling setting with another friend, and then leave the two children with toys while the sample is being tape recorded. If the child comes to the adult's setting, the sampler should appear to be doing some other activities (rather than just listening). This will often remove the authoritarian stress and allow the child to interact spontaneously with a peer.

When using the picture material, the sampler must remember that the goal of the language sample is to obtain a spontaneous and representative sample and not to play or to look at pictures. An idea that has to be prompted with comments like "Tell me more about the pictures" will not be spontaneous. If a child appears to have nothing to say about the pictures, then the child is finished with that sampling material. When the child is through, find another picture or another kind of sampling activity rather than push and restrict the language. During this period of sampling, the adult should be willing to talk about topics that emerge from ideas related to the pictures. For example, suppose the child says, "Oh, we have one of these at home." If the adult is too attached to the picture, he or she may forget to allow for spontaneity. The child's utterance about having one at home introduces a conversational topic the adult should encourage by commenting or saying, for example, "Oh, tell me about it" or "You do?" or "At *your* home?"

Following these suggestions is more likely to yield a spontaneous and representative language sample. There are additional suggestions for obtaining language samples in the literature (Lee, 1974; Longhurst, 1974; Wilson, 1969). The two key considerations are these: (1) the sample must be representative; and (2) the sample must be spontaneous. Both of these conditions necessitate appropriate contexts for collecting the samples.

Goals for Qualitative Analysis

A qualitative analysis of a language sample attempts to answer questions that are not answered by methods previously described or by present standardized tests. These questions are aimed at determining the child's semantic and pragmatic abilities and include the following:

1. Does the child's language contain objects, actions, and events in a variety of relationships?
2. Does the child use a variety of forms to express a variety of functions? (Forms in this sense means different lexical terms and not necessarily forms of construction.)
3. Does the child use utterances that are appropriate for the context?
4. Does the child answer questions appropriately or does the child only respond?
5. Does the child initiate or create new utterances in new contexts?
6. Does the child use the same construction over and over with some of the same lexical terms?

7. Does the child exhibit any of the specific language disorders described in the last chapter?
8. Does the child, in essence, perform a variety of speech acts?
9. Does the child use a variety of terms to denote space, time, quantity, and/ or does the child use a variety of qualifiers?

QUALITATIVE SEMANTIC AND PRAGMATIC ANALYSIS

Each of the questions about a child's semantic and pragmatic development will be discussed as it relates to segments of language samples obtained from children of various chronological ages and levels of language acquisition.

Language Sample 1

This first sample was obtained from a five-year, six-month-old female. The utterances were consecutive and taken from the middle of the sampling period (the period believed to be the most representative portion). The sample was taken in the context of free play with the objects in a doll house while the adult sampler followed the child's language leads.

> Child: "Where's the other one of these?" *(These* refer to a piece of furniture.)
> Adult: "I don't know."
> Child: "Did you lost it?"
> Adult: "I don't think so."
> Child: "Maybe you did."
> Adult: "Maybe."
> Child: "Then she fell down." (The doll fell out of the kitchen chair.)
> Adult: (No response.)
> Child: "Well, at least we still got some more chairs to eat with."
> Adult: "Uh, huh."
> Child: "Now they can eat." (All of the dolls are seated except Dad.)
> Adult: "Good."
> Child: "The Dad's gonna watch it."
> Adult: "Okay."
> Child: "The sister's gonna sit here."
> Adult: "Okay."
> Child: "The mother's gonna be cooking dinner if I can ever get her in this squishy house."
> Adult: "Okay."
> Child: "I have to get out this stuff." (Child removes excess furniture from the house.)

Adult: "Uh, huh."
Child: "I guess she's gonna go up and take a rest." (The sister is
walked up the stairs to the bedroom.)
Adult: "Okay."

The child's body orientation, eye contact, and prosodic features were appropriate for all utterances. (Observational information will be considered later in
this chapter.) The child's utterances may be used as a basis for asking the questions regarding semantic and pragmatic development. Although a minimum of
fifty utterances is usually considered representative, only eleven utterances will
be considered here for ease in illustrating specific language skills. For this
child, the rest of the sample indicated that these eleven utterances were typical.
The following questions and answers are necessary for a qualitative analysis of
the semantic and pragmatic skills:

1. *Does the child's language contain objects, actions, and events in a variety of relationships?* Yes, objects and people are used as initiators of
   action ("she's gonna" or "you lost") as well as recipients of action
   ("cooking dinner" or "take a little rest") and as part of different events
   ("dinner," "rest," "lost," "fell down," etc). Remember that this
   child's language cannot be described by simple semantic relational rules.
   If one wanted to write the grammar according to the function of the words
   in the construction, then a case grammar would be used (see Chafe, 1970;
   Fillmore, 1968).

2. *Does the child use a variety of forms to express a variety of functions?*
   Yes. The child used two types of question forms ("Did . . . " "Where
   . . . ") as well as declarative forms. In other segments of the sample, the
   child also used imperative forms ("Bring it out here . . . "). The functions include finding out information ("Where's . . . "); making a comment ("Maybe you did"); declaring or reporting ("Now they can do it");
   stating information ("Then she fell down"); and explaining ("If I can
   ever get in this squishy house").

3. *Are the child's utterances appropriate for the context?* Yes. The referents
   were appropriate for the situation, and the child waited for the adult's utterances and then continued with the same topic.

4. *Does the child answer questions appropriately or does she only respond?*
   Within the eleven utterances, there is no direct answer to this question.
   There is an indirect answer, however. The child asked, "Did you lost it?"
   and the adult said, "I don't think so." The child removed "think" and
   said, "Maybe you did." In other segments of the sample, the child answered the questions appropriately. Since the adult sampler should be following the child's language lead, in another portion of the evaluation the

adult will want to ask specific questions in order to determine if the child can answer questions that require following and attending to the speaker's specific referents.

5. *Does the child initiate or create new utterances in new contexts?* Yes. This child was creating new contexts such as "cooking" or "resting," and the utterances were spontaneous and novel.

6. *Does the child use forms that are rigid?* The only rigidity in this sample was the phrase "well at least . . . " which was used four times in seventy-five utterances. It is interesting that this stylistic variation, certainly not a problem, was also observed with some frequency in the parent's language.

7. *Does the child exhibit any specific language disorders?* No. The use of "lost" for "lose" was an error in forming the past tense of an irregular verb; this is not a disorder but actually indicates change and growth in a child's language. The unusual construction " . . . we still got some more chairs to eat with" was not that semantically inappropriate in the context of the child trying to find enough chairs for all of the people at the table.

8. *Does the child perform a variety of speech acts?* Yes. This point is partially answered by the first three questions. The child is meeting the essential elements of specific speech acts and thus is effectively communicating a variety of ideas.

9. *Does the child use a variety of terms to denote time, space, quantity, and/ or does the child use a variety of qualifiers?* Yes. Time is expressed in the present ("we still have"), past tense ("did lost"), and future tense ("gonna be"). Quantity is expressed by terms such as "one of these" and "some more," as well as by the correct marking of nouns as singular or plural. Simple spatial terms denoting place ("get out" or "gonna go up") and qualifiers such as "squishy," "this stuff," "a little" were used.

The answers to these questions indicate that this child's semantic and pragmatic language skills are appropriate for effective communication. A quantitative analysis and the results of a comprehension test for vocabulary, syntax, and morphology indicated that this child was functioning at chronological age level (five years, six months). The conclusion is that the child is neither language delayed nor disordered in the development and use of specific language skills.

Language Sample 2

The next three segments were obtained from an eleven-year-old male. The first segment was in response to the question, "What did you do this morning?"

"Um well, the first time the first thing I did today was um well the first thing, well today the first thing I was went out to my first recess. Not my first recess, it wasn't a, it wasn't a school recess, it was just right before school started, cause if it was the first recess then I would have been tremendously late. Um and so it started from that and we came up and and then . . . different-like we came, well, one things we do is we came up and said things like, oh yea what was the next discussion on."

The second segment was typical of this child's attempt to converse spontaneously.

Question: "You get up at seven o'clock, right?"
Answer: "Normally, I don't get up at seven o'clock, but I did get up this morning."
Question: "What did you do after you got up?"
Answer: "Let's see, for the last few days I have . . . "
Question: "What did you do after you got up?"

The third segment was obtained when the adult asked the child, "What would you do at the store?"

"I don't know, I haven't looked over there. Um, not directly you know I haven't looked all over. Um, um the reason I have twenty some dollars is because see um, I see, I don't, of course, I don't get paid anything if, I um, don't work for anything, you know. Um which I think I would be kind of spoiled to get something just without work. And so I, so I um, um, so I well, um, what happens is, you would normally think at first that a route was fun. It isn't fun when you get used to it, you know for a little while. Um, so, so, what I did, I get, I help Mary Ellen on, on the certain part of the route . . . only do certain ones like now I do, used to do, etc., etc. . . . but it's just like a hill because a big hill would be a mountain . . . um well there's this hill it's long but it isn't it isn't big, you know . . . "(He never closes any topic. Finally he says) "We first started out on the paper route didn't we?" (He goes back to Mary Ellen and in two utterances is talking about hills again).

As might be discerned through a structural analysis, these three segments had adequate development of structural complexity for communication. According to the child's teacher, the boy's reading comprehension and understanding of academic tasks is fair and the child has passed public school speech and language screening for four years. The classroom teacher did think the child should see a psychologist, and the psychologist did enroll the child in counseling sessions. However, many of the child's problems are revealed in a semantic and pragmatic qualitative analysis of the child's language. Again the analysis is based on the same nine questions.

1. *Does the child's language contain objects, actions, and events in a variety of relationships?* Not really. This question cannot be answered clearly until the referents are considered. In other words, why does the child begin utterances that he cannot complete? Notice that the majority of utterances begin with initiators of action even though there are few recipients. One is led to wonder about this child's expression of *relationships*. It is the absence of a variety of these relationships that is suspect until other questions are asked.

2. *Does the child use a variety of forms to express a variety of functions?* This child does use questions and declarative forms, but the variety of functions must be evaluated. The intent of this boy's utterances is seldom clear to the hearer. Why are the referents unclear?

3. *Are the child's utterances appropriate to the context?* To answer this question, look at the topic and also at the way the utterances follow one another. For example, in the question-and-answer segment, the child is on the right topic (time), but when asked a specific question ("What did you do after you got up?") his utterance ("Let's see, for the last few days I have . . . ") did not satisfy the hearer. So the hearer interrupted for clarification. The child's utterances are topical but not referentially specific enough to be truly appropriate to the context.

4. *Does the child answer questions appropriately or does he only respond?* It's obvious to the hearer that this child is trying to answer the question but does not have the linguistic skills. It was indicated earlier that the child's syntax and morphology were adequate. The child's phonology is not a problem. This means the problem is in the semantic and pragmatic areas of language. It's obvious that the child is trying to answer the questions, because he has a continuous flow of conversation about the topic until the hearer interrupts to let the child know that enough information has been given or at least uttered. Only when the question requires a specific, often rehearsed, answer (such as "What did you have in your lunch?" "A sandwich"), does the boy stop with an immediate, specific answer. Although this child is trying to answer questions, his responses are not very effective in communicating his intent, partially because of the lack of specific referents as determined by the second question.

5. *Does the child initiate or create new utterances or new contexts?* Yes, he has the creativity but not the skills to express his ideas. The creativity is

apparent in his attempt to tell the hearer about his own experiences, but his constructions are poorly executed.

6. *Does the child use forms that are rigid?* He doesn't use the exact same sentences or phrases in a repetitive manner, but he uses *fillers* to replace referents he can't use. Examples of the fillers include: interjections (such as "um," "well," "so"); use of second person plural pronouns in a generic sense ("you . . . "); and use of phrases (such as "not directly," "well sort of" and "so forth"). These forms are rigid only in the sense that they add nothing to the language content and reduce the flexibility of the language and the power of the message.

7. *Does the child exhibit any specific language disorders?* After answering the first six questions, it should be apparent that this child's language is not semantically or pragmatically appropriate for effective communication. This indicates the presence of some specific problems specifying referents, which is suggestive of language disorders. The absence of specific referents coupled with the excessive use of fillers results in the hearer having difficulty following the child's intent and indicates that the child does not have a systematic development of language skills. One method of analysis is to list the specific disorders and check the sample for evidence of each type of problem.

a. *Auditory misperception.* None in these segments.

b. *Off target responding.* The sampler would have to ask the child a few more questions to determine if this problem exists. The child's answers to the questions indicate that the child cannot scan the previous question, determine the appropriate referent, and then comment on it. Therefore, it does seem that the child responds off target.

c. *Syntactic errors.* The child's utterances are often incomplete and/or redundant. For example, "The first time, the first thing I did . . . " illustrates the child's use of "first" in two adjacent phrases that are also redundant constructions. In this case, as in most samples that the author has analyzed, these syntactical (morphological) errors do have a semantic basis. If the child could specify the referent, the need for both phrases would be eliminated. In other conversations, this child sometimes had the recipient of action doing the action because he had reversed the structural component, direct objects, and subjects. For example, "The ball, uh, threw, the second base man."

The child's syntactic errors indicate a lack of understanding of the sequence of events as marked by linguistic forms. The idea of sequence of events being a semantic concern in these syntactic errors will be more obvious later in the qualitative analysis.

d. *Semantic word errors.* These errors are evident in this child's language—particularly with verbs that denote time, with space markers (such as "over there" being used to mean "here," and with "hill" and "mountain" being unclear referents because of the qualifier "big"). The difficulty with time markers is indicated by the confusion of "first" or "a few days" when the referent called for a specific time, and with "tremendously late" used as a phrase to explain "how late." If the child's language demonstrates semantic word errors with space and time markers, then the child is experiencing a disorder related to the development of space and time concepts. This specific type of language disorder is discussed in detail in Chapter 6.

For the present it should be noted that the sequencing problem suggested by unusual syntax is probably a symptom of the child's inability to organize the world with spatial and temporal linguistic markers. Further evidence for this type of problem consists of behavioral observations and teachers' anecdotal records that indicate that the child is seldom punctual, that he cannot follow verbal directions but can comprehend and answer questions at age level, and that he plays baseball and has other extracurricular activities typical of his age level but cannot accurately describe the sequence of activity for an event.

e. *Word finding difficulties.* Although this child experiences difficulty using words to specify an event, the problem does not appear to be one of recall but one of matching lexicon with the appropriate event. However, there is some indication that the child does have problems recalling nouns since there are a lot of indefinite fillers (such as "something," "it," "certain part," "just") in place of words with definite or referential meaning. Even the use of definite meanings is a problem since this child's referential clarity is not very good.

f. *Topic or referent identification.* This has already been determined to be part of the overall language problem. The child cannot identify the referent in the adult's questions, nor can he identify the referent within his own language.

g. *Neologisms.* Not present in these segments.

h. *Topic closure.* Topic closure is a problem for this child. Once the child begins to talk, he continues until the hearer indicates nonverbally or verbally that the child had said enough. Notice that the child repeats ideas. This is typical of a topic closure problem which is often linked with a child's inability to scan and determine the referent. This child continues talking because he cannot identify what has been said nor that the information has communicated the intended message.

Another indication of a topic closure problem, related to an inability to scan the contextual message for a referent, is evidenced during the question-and-answer segment. The child's utterance, "Let's see, for the last few days I have . . . " is really part of his previous utterance,

"... but I did get up this morning ...." During this segment the child is not aware of the interruption by the hearer nor is he aware of the original question, "What did you do after you got up?" The child is talking but isn't sure what is being said, so he continues until something or someone stops him.

i. *Tangentiality.* Tangentiality often occurs when a child can't use the appropriate referent and can't determine when he's said enough. Consequently, one idea leads to another idea. In this case the topic of the store leads to the topic of the paper route, then to the idea of hills and mountains, and so forth. This child even recognizes the tangentiality because he says, "We first started out on the paper route."

j. *Echolalia, verbal perseveration, and phonological disorders.* Not present in this sample.

8. *Does the child perform a variety of speech acts?* The purpose or intention behind some of his statements is not clear because the proposition or content of the utterance does not specify the referents. The child is obviously attempting to perform a variety of speech acts but is ineffective because of the presence of language disorders.

9. *Does the child use a variety of terms to denote time, space, quantity, and/ or does the child use a variety of qualifiers?* Yes, the child uses a variety of these terms, but the concepts do not show a high level of semantic development.

In conclusion, the qualitative analysis of this child's language sample shows that he exhibits a general language disorder as evidenced by specific problems with semantic word errors, identification of the referents, tangential phrasing, and topic closure problems. These specific problems are linked to the child's inability to properly organize space and time by use of linguistic terms. The reader is encouraged to go back to the beginning of this section and reread the child's three language segments to pick out these problems.

Language Sample 3

This next sample is too short to draw any conclusions about the child's overall language skills, but the segment does illustrate some specific skills.

Adult: "Tell me about this picture."
Child: "Sleeping."
Adult: "And?"
Child: "Tying his boot."
Child: "There two mouse."

Adult: "What about this one?"
Child: "I can't know."
Child: "That mouse."
Adult: (turn page)
Child: "I can't know."
Adult: "Tell me about this one."
Child: "Let's see."
Child: "He's going to hide in the box."
Adult: "And this one."
Child: "I can't know."
Child: "I don't want to read some more."
Adult: "What do you want to talk about?"
Child: "I like puppies."
Adult: "Do you have a puppy?"
Child: "Yea, we got a Fifi."
Adult: "Is he your puppy?"
Child: "Yea."
Adult: "What does she look like?"
Child: "Kind of like that one except she all white."
Adult: "She looks like this one?"
Child: "All of these don't like Fifi." (referring to spots on the dog in the picture)
Adult: "The dogs don't like her."
Child: "Fifi's all white."
Adult: "Oh, they don't look like her."
Child: "Just a little tiny dog."
Adult: "She's a tiny dog."
Child: "Like that."

The context for these utterances was a storybook that the child had chosen, but then the child switched to spontaneous conversation. The age of the eleven-year-old male in Sample 2 was not that important because he was really beyond the seven- to eight-year-old plateau, but in this sample the age is significant. This child is five years, ten months. Based on milestone data, the child's structural development is obviously delayed if this segment is representative of his true language abilities. These utterances were in fact typical of his best productions at any given time on any given day. Since age is important here and since the constructions are so simple, each of the constructions will be discussed and then the questions asked.

The first utterance, "sleeping," although a verb form, is functioning as a label of an event, action, or object. *Labeling* is a primitive type of function in which children are tagging an entire event with a linguistic unit. The unit may be a word, a phrase, or sentence, but the purpose does not alter or change the attitudes, beliefs, or behaviors of the hearer. Labels are often taught at the expense of more pragmatic language.

The second utterance, "tying his boot," is still not much more than a label, but the child should be given some credit for showing some semantic relationships. The phrase "I can't know" constituted at least half of the utterances in the entire sample. The use of "can't" is not a usual form, but the fact that the utterance is a rigid and overused form is of more significance.

The utterance "that mouse" is again a label. But this is followed by "let's see," which is a request to see. The child then says, "I don't want to read some more," which is a functional utterance and an indication of the child's competence if the language is pragmatic. The conversation that follows is the most representative in the sample because the child is talking spontaneously and the utterances are part of the performed speech acts.

The utterance "I like puppies" is stimulated by the picture of dogs in the storybook. The child then answers a question with more information than requested. Notice the use of "a" before "Fifi" which makes the hearer believe that Fifi might be an object even though the topic is "dogs." In the next utterance, "kind of like that one except she all white," the child uses the picture to assist in communicating his idea that Fifi is like the dog in the picture but Fifi is all white.

Because the child lacks linguistic skills, the child says "All of these don't like Fifi," which has an entirely different meaning than "These dogs don't look like Fifi," which is also very different from "Fifi doesn't have all of these spots." The last utterance is probably what the child meant, since the dogs in the picture had spots and the child followed the previous utterance with "Fifi's all white." The child doesn't follow the adult's utterance but continues to talk about the picture with "just a little tiny dog." He then points to a small dog and says, "like that."

Now that each utterance has been separately considered, it should be easier to answer the questions:

1. *Does the child's language contain objects, actions, and events in a variety of relationships?* From this limited segment, it appears that the child's ability to express these relationships is limited even though he apparently understands a variety of semantic relationships.

2. *Does the child use a variety of forms to express a variety of functions?* Again, from this limited segment that is typical of the entire sample, it appears that the forms are quite restricted and that the functions are also limited. Restricted forms mean that the child's ability to use syntax and morphology for expressing ideas is limited.

If the answers to the first and second questions were grouped, one might conclude that this child has developed adequate semantic concepts but that the form for expression has not paralleled this development. But the functions are also limited, and complex linguistic forms are needed to express a variety of functions. From clinical studies and observations it appears that *a child who doesn't develop a variety of functions appears to have difficulty with developing the forms for expression.* This statement is supported by some intervention research (Lucas & Hoag, 1976; Lucas, 1977; Mundell & Lucas, 1978) that illustrates that teaching functional language develops syntactical and morphological complexity, whereas programs that emphasize structure for some of the same children do not facilitate function. Furthermore, literature regarding normal development (as cited in the first two chapters) suggests that a variety of functions may be expressed even prelinguistically by infants, suggesting that function precedes structure.

3. *Are the child's utterances appropriate to the context?* Yes and no. The child does stay on the topic, but he manipulates the topic so that the appropriateness is dependent on his own language production. This is typical of a very young child who is socially involved more with himself than with others; it's not typical of a five-year, ten-month-old child.

4. *Does the child answer questions appropriately or does he just respond?* Yes, when he knows the answer or wishes to respond, he does answer appropriately within his level of comprehension and within his range of linguistic skills.

5. *Does the child initiate or create new utterances in new contexts?* Although many of the child's utterances are novel except for the rigid form "I can't know," the contexts are limited or rigid; that is, the child maintains the contexts specific to what he can talk about.

6. *Does the child use forms that are rigid?* Yes, as previously discussed.

7. *Does the child exhibit any specific language disorders?* The only obvious errors are connected to the child's inability to use the semantic concepts in a conventional manner. This problem results in the syntactic and semantic word problems that were discussed in the analysis of the individual utterances.

8. *Does the child perform a variety of speech acts?* No. The child does attempt to influence the hearer's behavior, attitudes, or beliefs in a variety of ways. But because the child has difficulty with the propositional content and the essential rule, his attempts are often incomplete. Remember, performing a speech act is an active process. The child is either effective or ineffective; that is, the child either performs or does not perform the speech act. According to this standard this child does not perform a vari-

ety of speech acts. His language usage skills must be considered minimally effective.

9. *Does the child use a variety of terms to denote time, space, quantity, and/ or does the child use a variety of qualifiers?* The child does use simple qualifying and quantifying terms, sometimes in a redundant or inappropriate way. His use of space and time is limited to the use of early developing concepts such as "in," "up," and "down."

From this qualitative language analysis, it appears that this child may have a pragmatic language disorder that manifests itself in a semantic inability and includes morphological and syntactic problems, resulting in an overall delay of language development. This conclusion would be verified or rejected on the basis of other test results and behavioral observations. Even though the forms of expression are delayed, the product is a language disorder. The child is not acquiring the semantic rules for pragmatic development.

Language Sample 4

This next segment was provided by a public school speech and language clinician who was keenly aware of the consequences of teaching structure at the expense of semantic and pragmatic skills. The clinician had attempted to give the *Northwest Syntax Screening Test* (Lee, 1971), but the child did not understand the task and so talked about the pictures. The clinician decided to listen to the child rather than stop the talking. Since test materials should not be used to elicit language samples and because the pictures are also limited in subject matter, the sample cannot be considered representative. However, the segment is included to illustrate some specific concerns regarding language development and intervention. The child is talking freely and the clinician is listening.

1. "This is a man is throwing to the ball."
2. "This is a boy not looking his ball."
3. "This is a boy found his ball."
4. "This is a girl got more two dogs."
5. "This is a boy wearing not mask."
6. "This is a cat yes playing."

The child's entire sample illustrated the same problem found in the first six utterances—namely, that the utterance always begins with a "This is ... " followed by a content utterance. Even though this segment is not considered representative, these types of utterances are also used by the child in spontaneous conversation. This sample warrants a few comments before answering the basic questions.

The first utterance, "This is a man is throwing to the ball" should have been either "The man is throwing the ball" or "The man is catching the ball." This child has been on a program to learn "This is a . . . ", and the programming has interfered with the child's acquisition of semantic relations. Therefore, the intent is not communicated because the child has been restricted to specific structures. The other structure that appears in an unnatural manner is the present progressive verb form ("is" + "-ing"). The child has also gone through a program for learning that construction.

The programming of structure at the expense of semantic and pragmatic skills need not be so obvious. One clinician did not realize the effects of her programs until she saw a child in the school hall and asked him about the day. The child said, "This is a pant—I have a blue." The child had on a new pair of blue pants. It would have been more meaningful and certainly more natural to say, "See, blue pants!" accompanying the utterance with appropriate non-verbal behavior and natural prosodic features. Although the construction would have been at a lower level, the utterance would have expressed good semantic relations. *If the semantic relations are not fostered, the subsequent reduction of the child's development of more advanced linguistically bound concepts restricts further cognitive or linguistic development.*

As a language consultant to schools and institutions, the author finds that it is almost always obvious what structures are being drilled in the child's therapy. For example, on one occasion when a child was talking spontaneously about many ideas, the adult sampler said, "Now, what's happening in this picture, James?" The child picked up on the author's utterance as a stimulus cue from therapy and said, "The boy *is* jumping" with very unnatural prosody. *Whenever the structures are unnatural, the prosodic features are unnatural, and the intent of the utterance is impaired. Thus the sincerity rule is questioned.*

Most clinicians who see Language Sample 4 immediately analyze the length and the word classes without looking at the content. Consequently these clinicians conclude that the child has fairly good language skills. The clinician who had worked with this child had made an effort to facilitate the child's semantic and pragmatic skills while alleviating the stereotyped structures. The clinician found that the child's competent language level was typically three to four words long which was sufficient to express a variety of semantic relations such as "My doll sits here" or "The man throw ball" or "The buggy goes too." If the reader looks back at the language sample, this natural language ability can be recognized in the comment or content portion of the utterances (that is, the sentence portion that follows the *"This is . . ."*). The child is capable of predicating and producing a proposition.

Notice that when the child feels forced to use a specific structure, not only do the semantic relations become unclear because of the unusual word ordering but the acquisition of functors such as "not" or "the" is confusing since there is no natural place to put these words.

The basic questions may be answered. The reader is encouraged to try to answer the questions before looking at the written answer.

1. *Does the child's language contain action, objects, and events in a variety of relations?* The objects, actions, and events are present, but because the child is trying to plug ideas into nonfunctional structures, the relations are unclear.

2. *Does the child use a variety of forms to express a variety of functions?* Definitely not. The child's natural role system has been disrupted.

3. *Are the child's utterances appropriate for the context?* Since the child was not flexible in the setting, a different sample is required to answer this question. A flexible setting or context would encourage the most representative and spontaneous sample.

4. *Does the child answer questions appropriately or does he just respond?* In trying to get the child to follow directions, he did not answer questions very well. However, more sampling would be required before these results are deemed conclusive. The child may have been conditioned to the presence of the language clinician and thus performs only as previous language sessions had dictated.

5. *Does the child initiate or create new utterances in new contexts?* This is an important question for this child. He did not use his language in new contexts until after the stereotyped utterances were eliminated. Then the child not only initiated and created new utterances, but the language was very functional. This suggests that inappropriate intervention actually restricted language development and therefore created a language disorder.

6. *Does the child use forms that are rigid?* Yes! With language that is flexible, one has the power to meet one's needs in a variety of new settings, whereas rigid language limits one's ability to develop more language to meet new needs.

7. *Does the child exhibit any specific language disorders?* This is a difficult question to answer for this specific child. The child's language forms and intended message are quite unusual, but this segment doesn't really assess what the child is acquiring. The segment represents what the child has learned. The learned constructions represent a disorder fostered in the child by the clinician or educator who taught these forms. The unusual patterns may not even show up in a more spontaneous sample obtained after the stereotyped constructions are eliminated. On the other hand, the child's language may show specific problems even after the stereotyped utterances are eliminated, due to the natural processes being affected.

8. *Does the child perform a variety of speech acts?* No. If the child's message is ineffective for a variety of reasons—because of unclear intent, or because of problems in expressing the proposition, and/or because of the problems with the essential elements such as prosodic features—then speech acts are not being completed.
9. *Does the child use a variety of terms to denote time, space, quantity, and/ or does the child use a variety of qualifiers?* Even though the segment content is limited by the subject matter available in the pictures, it usually happens that when a child's structures are linguistically limited, the development of cognitive concepts related to quantity, space, and/or time will also be limited.

Conclusions regarding this child's specific language skills must be considered tentative until a truly representative sample can be obtained.

Language Sample 5

The next sample is from a six-year-old male who is looking at a storybook about a family of bears who try to get honey but are chased by bees. The clinician's comments were noncommittal and followed the child's lead.

1. "Who's in the tree?"
2. "Oh, oh he water."
3. "Who fall in that?"
4. "That's his coppee."
5. "He—"(pause) "He's pouring the coppee in the cup, more gone."
6. "Boy—"(pause)"—eats the coppee."
7. "A house—"(pause)"—light." (There's assumed to be a house in the tree).
8. "Who's—"(pause) "He's run." (The bear was running).
9. "Who's that doing?"
10. "Honey."
11. (The boy bear was following the daddy bear on the road). "Boys put the foots and his toe, see."
12. "On he's . . . he put his tree" (possibly "three") "foots."
13. "He's sawn the butterfly." (bees)
14. "He flowed away and its butterfly."
15. "See de de de" (pointed to the three bees).
16. "He's taking the hand." (The boy bear is holding daddy bear's hand.)
17. "Oops! He's sweet the butterfly."

18. "Climbing."
19. "He's climbing the ground." (a hill)
20. "Who's on the match?" (a bee on the flower)
21. "A match."
22. (The clinician said, "That's a flower.") He said, "Flower?"
23. "See."
24. "Flying the tree?"
25. "Who's fall the bee?" (The daddy bear was reaching into a tree, and it looked like he was going to fall.)
26. "Who's fall?"
27. "Wait! That's an owl!"
28. "He's tryin' go bye bye."
29. "He's go bye bye."
30. "See go bye bye."
31. "See thats trees."
32. "Goed away."
33. "He's took a mouth and climbs."
34. "He's took a teeth and he bite—"(pause)"—over the key."
35. "Where's the flies?" (Clinician asked, "Where's the what?")
36. "Butterflies in the door."
37. "Who's bumped it?"
38. "Who's bumped?"
39. "That's a tree."
40. "He's go away in the butterfly."
41. "He's bye bye."
42. "Boy bye."
43. "Boy."
44. "He's giving the hand and bang."
45. "Wait! He's falled the lap."
46. "Look butterfly!"
47. "Goes in the bucket and the tree."
48. "Who's in the coffee? Huh?"
49. "In the coffee."

This sample will be analyzed by the standard questions. It's obvious that the child has a language problem, but the specific problems would not be determined by a quantitative or structural language analysis.

1. *Does the child's language show a variety of agents, actions, and events in a variety of relations?* The utterances certainly contain objects and actions to describe events, but some of the semantic relations are unusual. For example, utterance 24 *("Flying the tree?")* has the tree flying, which

was not semantically correct and would, under most circumstances, be quite extraordinary. In utterance 17 *("He's sweet the butterfly")*, "sweet" is used in a verb position, which results in an unusual relationship between "sweet" and "butterfly" ("He's sweet butterfly"— actually the insect was a bee).

2. *Does the child use a variety of forms to express a variety of functions?* The child is definitely having problems expressing his ideas. The utterances are poorly formed even though it's apparent that the child is trying to express a variety of functions such as asking for information, describing, making requests, etc. Therefore, the child's pragmatic skills are more appropriate than his semantic abilities are. It's quite unusual to have better pragmatic skills than semantic skills, though for this child, the weakness in semantic skills is not pervasive (as might be initially expected) but very specific. This point will be further discussed in a subsequent question.

3. *Are the child's utterances appropriate for the context?* Yes, the context and utterances match well, but some of the utterances appear to contain words that the child doesn't intend to use or words that do not match the topic in the picture. For example, the clinician repeatedly modeled the lexical term, "bees," even though the child continued to call the bees "butterflies" because the picture depicted wings and showed the insect flying. Wings is a perceptual attribute and flying is a functional attribute that the child has narrowly associated to the term "butterflies." This is a classic semantic word error. The child's ability to sort the semantic features in the environment is not adequate to learn concepts as readily as is expected of a child this age.

4. *Does the child answer questions appropriately or does the child just respond?* The child attempts to answer questions in which the answer is specific—that is, in which the referent is clearly a given object or person.

5. *Does the child initiate or create new utterances in new contexts?* The child has a problem specifying the referents (for example, "butterflies" for "bees") in the contexts, but the child does initiate and create new utterances.

6. *Does the child use forms that are rigid?* The child does not use stereotyped utterances, but the high content and low structural skills might suggest some problems with acquiring the rules for form, unless there is some underlying semantic problem.

7. *Does the child exhibit any specific language disorders?* By now, the reader should be familiar with the specific language disorders presented in this book. So instead of going through the list of disorders, the reader should try to spot the disorders by looking at the sample. For example, in utterance 4 the child says "coppee" for "coffee." The clinician said

"coffee," but the child continued to say "coppee," even though the child used other f's and p's in all word positions in other parts of the language sample. Furthermore, the standard articulation test revealed no errors. Therefore, the child must be misperceiving the specific word; "coppee" could be considered an auditory misperception. Other examples include "tree" for "three" and "de, de, de" for counting out three "bees."

One of the most glaring characteristics of this child's language sample is the unusual use of certain words such as "climbing the ground." This semantic word error is a classic example of a spatial problem. The reader might ask, "Why isn't it just a misuse of a word? Why does it necessarily represent a spatial problem?" There are other examples that support the spatial problem hypothesis. In utterance 16, the child uses "taking" (action of receiving) instead of a word such as "*holding*" in reference to a position. The use of "match" for "flower" in utterance 20 suggests an inability to spatially organize a pattern into a perceived gestalt. The child sees the stem and not the petals, nor does the child relate to other perceptual or functional attributes in the rest of this picture or in the other pictures. For example, in utterance 26 the child asks, "Who's fall . . . ?" when it is obvious from the picture that the Daddy bear will fall. In utterance 33, the child's statement, "He took a mouth and climbs," would be meaningless unless the context is considered. The picture showed an animated drawing of a boy running with his mouth open and his arms outstretched. Since the boy had not had his mouth open in the picture on the opposite page, the child thought the boy had taken a mouth; and since there was no ground drawn for spatial reference, the boy's raised leg meant that he was climbing. Obviously the child was not putting objects, actions, and events into relationships that could then be expressed linguistically.

With spatial problems, the utterances that appear to be off target have a logical explanation based on the child's perception of the environment. Semantic word errors can also explain the syntactic errors in which the adjective is used as a verb (for example, "sweet") or the recipient of action should have been the actor. *If a child has difficulty attaching the lexicon to perceptions, and/or the perceptions as described by conventional lexicon are distorted, then structuring the semantic concepts by conventional forms may also be distorted.* In other words, if the underlying semantic relations are distorted, the surface representations may also be distorted.

Since the child is experiencing difficulty in putting semantic relations together into organized linguistic patterns, it is not unusual that the child is also experiencing difficulty identifying referents. The ability to attach the linguistic representation to an experience is closely related to the ability to identify the respective agents, actions, and objects in a referential manner. This child's language disorders might be summarized by saying that the child has difficulty representing perceptual and functional attributes with appropriate linguistic markers, resulting in semantic word errors, auditory misperceptions, and syntactic errors.

8. *Does the child use a variety of speech acts?* The child attempts a variety of functions, but the poor formulation (essential rules) of the content (propositional rule) results in incomplete performances of speech acts.

9. *Does the child use a variety of terms to denote space, time, quantity, and/ or does the child use a variety of qualifiers?* No. In fact, the attempt to use "in" was not successful. In utterance 40, "He's going away in the butterfly," should have been "They or the bees and he are going away." In utterance 47, ". . . *in the bucket"* referred to the bear looking into a hole in the tree. Apparently this child does not have a good enough grasp of the linguistic skills regarding his perceptions of space to adequately explain the situation. Even simple qualifiers are used sparingly.

The child is apparently experiencing difficulty acquiring semantic features for representing ideas in a conventional way. The lack of a semantic basis results in syntactic and semantic word errors. The auditory misperception is a key to the child's problem: auditory skills for comprehending the aural/oral system must be deviant, whereas the good pragmatic skills are indicative of a visual system that is intact.

This hypothesis was further substantiated by standardized tests, including a *Wechsler Intelligence Scale for Children* (Revised Edition, 1974), which indicated more than a 50-point discrepancy between the verbal tasks and the performance tasks. Since a 12-point difference is usually considered significant, this 50-point discrepancy was exceptional. The child's visual-motor strengths on the performance tasks aided the clinician in determining the therapeutic manner of material presentation, but the child's specific language problems may be best remediated by direct linguistic intervention tasks.

Summary

The use of a qualitative language analysis is necessary to determine a child's typical semantic and pragmatic skills. As the five segments from language samples illustrated, the child's semantic development and subsequent use is a critical part of the child's overall language abilities. These analyses helped clinicians identify several different pattern types with either a single disorder occurring or being combined with other deviations. Each child's language sample reflects one child's experiences and ability to deal with those experiences.

Language sample analyses provide a tremendous amount of information not only about the problems but also about why the problems exist. It also may be desirable to compare a child's overall performance to that of other children. A general profile of the child's abilities in other areas of development may be obtained from standardized tests in which data from a population determine a norm against which to compare a specific child's performance. There are many standardized or norm referenced tests in related areas of language development, particularly syntax and morphology. For a listing and review of these tests, see Darley (1979), Darley and Spriestersbach (1978), McLean and Snyder-McLean (1978), and Nation and Aram (1977).

Once the analyses are performed, the clinician should be able to plan for therapy. Understanding the child's ability to utilize certain types of information helps the clinician determine appropriate intervention. It is reasonable to assume that the child with a semantic language disorder has difficulty with auditory and/or visual processing skills. The types of utterances may be analyzed not only for disorders (auditory misperceptions, semantic word errors, etc.) but also for the logic of the uttered proposition. For example, why did the child say "climbing the ground"? The person in the picture was on hands and knees on the ground. The child's visual interpretation of the picture was correct, but the auditory attachment of signs and symbols was inappropriate. Another child thought the train coming out of the tunnel was different from the train going into the tunnel, even though the perceptual attributes were the same. Thus the child's visual perception was inaccurate, but his auditory attaching of the signs was adequate. In this case the child's semantic word errors were a product of his visual interpretation.

Standardized tests that assess processing skills should be able to support or reject the information generated by the language sample, and the qualitative analyses should be able to confirm or deny the validity of the data from the standardized test. Independent use of either standardized tests or the qualitative language sample is inadequate.

BEHAVIORAL OBSERVATIONS

How the child interacts with the environment provides the observer with significant information, confirms or rejects the inferences drawn from qualitative analysis of the language sample, and often suggests effective avenues for remediation. Therefore it is important to consider behavioral observations related to the specific language disorders and to the questions used to determine the child's general semantic and pragmatic language skills. The ultimate goal is a picture of the total child and thus the answer to the following question: "How do the qualitative analysis, behavioral observations, and standardized tests interact in diagnostic evaluations?" Some behavioral observations related to the previously described semantic disorders are reviewed, followed by a discussion of the behavioral observations that characterize a pragmatic disorder.

Semantic Disorders

stares at wall in thought.

The child with semantic difficulties often exhibits puzzled facial expressions, such as a raised brow or furrowed forehead perhaps because the child cannot express acquired knowledge or because the child is confused by the relationships among symbols that represent acquired knowledge.

The child's organizational problems can affect daily tasks or some motor tasks. For example, a child who plays the piano may easily memorize a piece of music but may have great difficulty learning the piece by following the visual music symbols. On the playground, a child may not understand directions or be able to conceptualize the purpose of a game without being walked through the game or verbalizing the sequence of events after the game. A child may begin to learn visual reading skills but then have trouble moving from sight vocabulary into sound blending or a phonics program. Similarly, a child may acquire basic numbers and the corresponding quantity concepts but not be able to do story problems or higher math problems. The child may show a lack of common sense or good judgment in everyday problem-solving skills because difficulty with semantic linguistic skills affects the child's ability to *use* language for thought. Conversely, a basic auditory inability to organize by linguistic skills also affects daily activities.

Some children with semantic language problems have been described as "lazy" or "noncooperative" because they do not respond to situational demands as expected. For example, most adults would think that a child who stands on clothes when told, "Go get on your clothes," is defiant or "acting out." There is a difference, however, between the child who is acting out and the child with the semantic language difficulties—namely, the degree of seriousness the latter child brings to problem-solving situations. Children with semantic language disorders will be totally and consistently serious until language and/or academic intervention is utilized.

Behavioral information can help clinicians determine the child's learning strategies. The following questions can be useful in organizing the observational material:

1. *When the child is speaking or attempting to communicate, does the child observe the hearer's face?* The child should glance at or make eye contact with the hearer so that when the roles are switched the child is able to follow the speaker's referent. Excessive observation indicates that the child needs the visual information to assist in following the speaker. For example, one child pulled on the hearer's sleeve to turn the speaker

around. This child needed maximum visual cues in order to determine if his speech was being understood. The child had a severe semantic language disorder that was best assisted by supplementing therapy with sign language. A child who seldom glances or makes eye contact with the hearer often exhibits problems with referent identification, topic closure, and echolalia.

2. *Can the child respond appropriately to a speaker while the child is engaged in play?* The child should be able to do another activity while talking. The child who is incoherent (particularly tangential and off topic) while playing, is probably having difficulty following the referent of the immediate environment while talking about a referent that may be absent or a topic that is removed. Thus the presence of visual referents may be necessary to this child's language skills.

3. *Do the child's language difficulties cross reading, writing, and speaking situations?* There are some children who do not acquire oral language but are capable of reading. Do not ignore the child's preference for a visual system of input; use the visual system to teach the child.

4. *What does the child do when watching television?* Does the child follow the action or story or does the child follow the faces? A child should be able to follow the story without needing visual cues from the speaker's face.

5. *What does the child do with a picture book?* Does the child go through the book looking at the pages in a systematic order (suggesting visual language), or does the child flip a couple of pages and then put the book down (suggesting that the picture sequence has little meaning)?

6. *Do the child's language skills, particularly phonology, improve when the child is looking at the speaker's mouth?*

7. *Does the child use body movement to manipulate the environment?* This particular observation is discussed further under pragmatic assessment, since the child who must use body movement to meet needs is having problems being an effective communicator.

8. *Does the child use an abundance of gesture or pantomime, indicating an understanding more of the environment through nonauditory means?*

9. *How do the significant people in the child's environment affect the child's linguistic and social behavior?* Does the child verbalize more or less with different people in different situations? What is the quality of the verbalization? When a child has semantic disorders that affect the pragmatic skills, then the presence of people in the child's immediate surroundings may affect these skills by generating stress, anxiety, or soothing effects.

10. *Does the child follow routine?* This question is particularly helpful in trying to ascertain whether the child is using referential meaning to fol-

low the topics of conversation and whether the child is having difficulty dealing with concepts of space, time, quantity, and quality.

Pragmatic Disorders

Whether or not a child is effective in conveying an intent determines the child's pragmatic competency. A child may be considered ineffective in performing speech acts when the child: (1) physically attempts to solve situational problems better suited to verbal solutions; (2) never initiates verbalizations to meet specific needs; (3) inappropriately cues the hearer with inadequate paralinguistic cues; and/or (4) lacks the ability to specify referents.

Examples of incomplete speech acts or ineffective pragmatic skills include the following:

- If the child consistently waits to be given materials, snacks, and toys rather than asks for them, particularly if the child is encouraged to request

- If the child makes utterances that are inappropriately stressed or are produced with insufficient intensity, observation, or eye contact to signal a hearer that the child is speaking

- If the child makes frequent utterances that lack referential clarity, so that the hearer expresses a lack of understanding

- If the child attempts to solve needs by getting out of a set, leaving a designated activity area, or by manipulating the situation aggressively or passively.

These behavioral observations suggest the presence of a semantic language disorder that negatively affects the child's usage of linguistic skills for effective communication. The result is a pragmatic disorder. Analysis of the qualitative language sample allows for a description of the child's skills and/or problems. The standardized measures support an analysis of the *overall* general language development, if the measures are content valid (see Chapter 9).

CRITERION REFERENCED MEASURES

The behavioral observations, qualitative language sample analysis, and standardized tests may also be coupled with or supplemented by criterion referenced measures. The criterion referenced tests compare the child's semantic and pragmatic skills with a criterion. This criterion is the knowledge that is available regarding normal sociolinguistic development. McLean and Snyder-McLean (1978) have described one type of criterion referenced measure, a "communication assessment profile" and sampling procedures for children who are acquiring language. The Behavioral Inventory of Speech Act Performances (BISAP) is also a criterion referenced measure that assesses how well a child can use the form of language, the meaning, and the paralinguistic features to be an effective performer of specific speech acts. The following section describes the BISAP and presents it more as a methodology consideration than as a specific instrument.

BISAP

The BISAP (Lucas, 1977) was based on an idea (Hoag, 1975) developed for use in a pilot therapy project (Lucas & Hoag, 1976) and then tested for its feasibility in assessing therapy gains (Lucas, 1977). Appendix A describes the limited statistical analysis that has been performed on the inventory to determine whether or not the criterion (normal children's use of speech acts in the same contexts) is a reliable and valid measure. The assessed speech act has been defined according to Searle's (1969) theorized preparatory, propositional, sincerity, and essential semantic rules described in Chapter 2. Since the rules constitute the speech act, the rules also provide the minimum requirements for a speech act in a predetermined context.

Scoring the performance of the speech act is accomplished by using a dichotomous yes/no checklist that indicates whether the child performed the essential element (yes) or did not perform the element (no). The scoring sheet (see Appendix B) shows those essential elements that determine whether or not the illocutionary force will probably affect the hearer as intended and therefore complete the speech act. Although it is recognized that other essential elements or illocutionary force devices may be operating to clarify the linguistic context, only those essential elements believed to be needed to affect a hearer in a predetermined context have been presented.

Two testers, preferably two adults, are required to administer the tasks. The first tester provides the rules for the context (for example, "Let's play ball. Sherrie has the ball.") and the child is expected to perform the necessary linguistic and paralinguistic acts to complete the situation. Once the contextual rules are given to the child, the child becomes the speaker and the second tester becomes a hearer. This second person (really a tester) must not be included in the providing of contextual rules so that the child thinks that the hearer does not know what to do (sincerity rule). The child, as a speaker, must affect the hearer by using the essential elements of the speech act to participate in the situation.

If the child does not effectively perform the speech act (affect the hearer in an appropriate fashion) within one minute or less, depending on the anxiety exhibited by the child, the hearer provides a response that completes the situation and allows for success in the testing context. The tester may reword the contextual rules so that the child understands the situation, but in rewording should offer no new information that will act as a cue for completion of the speech act. For example, "Let's play ball. Ms. Smith has the ball." A rewording without new information might be, "If you want to play ball, Ms. Smith knows how to get the ball." An example of a rewording that adds new information might be, "Let's play ball. *Ask* Ms. Smith for the ball." In this last rewording, the child was told what to do to get the ball; this was the purpose of the task.

The predetermined tasks used to provide a context for assessing the speech acts should be varied to meet the needs of the child. It is important to reemphasize that this is not a standardized measure, but a measure that compares the child to a criterion. Once the tasks have been selected, a few three-to-five-year-old children who do not exhibit language delays or language disorders, should be administered the tasks to determine whether or not the criteria are valid. The author has used art tasks (1977) as described in Appendix C, as well as preschool academic tasks and infant-to-caretaker physical needs tasks.

Several samples of children have been assessed for their use of speech acts. Included were samples of emotionally disturbed children, trainable and educable mentally retarded school-age children, Down's Syndrome infants, and upper and lower socioeconomic school-age children without language difficulties. As long as the tasks are based on the child's background of experiences, the BISAP is an effective criterion referenced measure. The clinician who uses the qualitative language sample analysis coupled with behavioral observation data and the results of the BISAP should have more than enough information to assess a child who is suspected of having a language disorder that affects pragmatic skills.

SUMMARY OF ASSESSMENT OF SEMANTIC LANGUAGE DISORDERS

As described in Chapters 1 and 2, the child's general cognitive and social levels are reflected by the semantic and pragmatic level of development. Assessment of semantic and pragmatic language must therefore consider the total child as he or she interacts in a context to affect a hearer's attitudes, beliefs, or behaviors. The effectiveness of the child's interactions is a function of the child's ability to map on structures to the cognitive basis for social use. More significantly, the ability to use the language also appears to influence the child's further language development. Therefore, a qualitative language analysis that considers the child's effectiveness in using linguistic skills to manipulate the environment is best considered when compared to the child's structural, morphophonemic development as measured by a variety of marketed, standardized tests.

It is not feasible to do extensive language sample analyses and a criterion referenced measure such as the BISAP on all children. In fact, the only reason to do the BISAP is if the child is exhibiting a possible pragmatic language disorder, and this can be determined through behavioral observations. The information from the BISAP will be useful in planning therapy (Chapter 8). Once the clinician becomes acquainted with the questions asked in the qualitative language analysis, these questions may be answered as the teacher or clinician is listening to the child. The results of this analysis can point to the need to do more assessment in a particular language area.

Questions

1. How do you determine whether a child has a problem with semantic word errors or with referent identification?
2. How do topic closure and topic identification relate to each other?
3. How does a qualitative language sample analysis influence the overall evaluation?
4. What variables influence obtaining a representative and spontaneous language sample?
5. What types of questions are asked to determine the quality of language obtained through sampling procedures?

REFERENCES

Brown, R. *A first language: The early stages.* Cambridge, Mass.: Harvard University Press, 1973.

Chafe, W. L. *Meaning and the structure of language.* Chicago, Ill.: The University of Chicago Press, 1970.

Crystal, D. *Working with LARSP.* New York: Elsevier, 1979.

Crystal, D., Fletcher, P., & Garman, M. *The grammatical analysis of language disability.* New York: Elsevier, 1976.

Darley, F. L. (Ed.). *Evaluation of appraisal techniques in speech and language pathology.* Reading, Mass.: Addison-Wesley Publishing Co., 1979.

Darley, F. L., & Spriestersbach, D. C. *Diagnostic methods in speech pathology* (2nd ed.). New York: Harper & Row, 1978.

Fillmore, C. J. The case for case. In E. Bach & R. T. Harms (Eds.), *Universals of linguistic theory.* New York: Holt, Rinehart, & Winston, 1968.

Hannah, E. P. *Applied linguistic analysis.* Northridge, Ca.: Joyce Motion Picture Co., 1974.

Hoag, L. *Application of speech act theory to language disordered children: The program.* Unpublished manuscript, University of Illinois, 1975.

Holland, A. L. Language therapy for children: Some thoughts on context and content. *Journal of Speech and Hearing Disorders,* 1975, *40,* 514-523.

Johnson, W., Darley, F. L., & Spriestersbach, D. C. *Diagnostic methods in speech pathology.* New York: Harper & Row, 1963.

Lee, L. *Northwest syntax screening test.* Evanston, Ill.: Northwestern University Press, 1971.

Lee, L. *Developmental sentence analysis: A grammatical assessment procedure for speech and language clinicians.* Evanston, Ill.: Northwestern University Press, 1974.

Longhurst, T. M. (Ed.). *Linguistic analysis of children's speech.* New York: MSS Information Corporation, 1974.

Lucas, E. V. The feasibility of speech acts as a language approach for emotionally disturbed children. (Doctoral dissertation, University of Georgia, 1977). *Dissertation Abstracts International,* 1978, *38,* 3479B-3967B. (University Microfilms, No. 77-30, 488).

Lucas, E., & Hoag, L. *Speech acts: A language therapy strategy for emotionally disturbed children.* Paper presented at the Interdisciplinary Linguistic Conference: Language Perspectives, Louisville, Kentucky, May 1976.

MacDonald, J. D., & Nikols, M. *Environmental language inventory.* Ohio State University: Nisonger Center, 1974.

McLean, J., & Snyder-McLean, L. *A transactional approach to early language training.* Columbus, Ohio: Charles E. Merrill, 1978.

Mundell, C., & Lucas, E. *A parent conducted pragmatic language program for Down's Syndrome Children.* An unpublished manuscript, Washington State University, 1978.

Nation, J. E., & Aram, D. M. *Diagnosis of speech and language disorders.* St. Louis, Mo.: CV Mosby Co., 1977.

Searle, J. R. *Speech acts: An essay in the philosophy of language.* Cambridge, England: Cambridge University Press, 1969.

Tyack, D. The use of language samples in a clinical setting. *Journal of Learning Disabilities,* 1973, *6,* 213-216.

Tyack, D., & Gottsleben, R. *Language sampling, analysis and training.* Palo Alto, Ca.: Consulting Psychologists Press, 1974.

Wechsler, D. *Manual for the Wechsler Intelligence Scale for Children—Revised.* New York: Psychological Corporation, 1974.

Wilson, M. E. A standardized method for obtaining a spoken language sample. *Journal of Speech and Hearing Research,* 1969, *12,* 95-102.

CHAPTER OBJECTIVES

- select tests that measure specific areas of language development.

- discuss the relationship of marketed tests to language sample results.

- demonstrate an ability to interpret the language test results.

- write the results of a language evaluation which includes standardized, formal, and informal measures.

- explain the process of hypothesis testing for selecting appropriate language tests.

- integrate standardized test results with language sample analyses or results.

- explain the different theoretical assumptions that underlie test purposes.

- recognize the difference between the results for a child with a language delay and a child with a language disorder.

- explain the relationship between the assessment of syntax, morphology, and semantics and pragmatics.

- explain how process testing is related to the assessment of linguistic abilities.

Chapter 5

Standardized Language Assessment and Evaluation

*A standard about the mean is simply a
deviation in a child's individuality!*

Chapter 4 discussed the assessment of semantic and pragmatic language disorders via formalized quantitative and qualitative measures. The purpose of this chapter is to suggest a method of total assessment that uses the results from marketed tests, language sample analyses, and behavioral observations.

DIAGNOSTIC ASSESSMENT FOR LANGUAGE

The purpose of diagnostic language testing is threefold: (1) to determine if the child has a language delay or language disorder; (2) to determine the child's level of language as compared to other children the same age; and (3) to determine the child's particular strengths in learning language so that an appropriate program of remediation may be developed.

Language Delay Versus Language Disorder

As discussed in Chapter 4, a child with a language delay will demonstrate an overall depression in language skills either in one linguistic area (such as syntax and morphology) or in all linguistic areas. Standardized tests are developed on the assumption that the child's development of language is orderly; any deviation from the normative pattern may be quantitatively measured. For example, if a six-year-old child performs at the four-year-old level on a test that assesses syntax and morphology, then the face value interpretation would be that the child's syntax and morphology are delayed two years.

A language disorder violates the basic assumption that language is developed in an orderly sequence. This violation threatens the validity of results that assume a comparison to normal development or normative data. Therefore, appropriate interpretation of the collective test results is even more important for the language disordered child than for the language delayed child. For example, suppose a seven-year-old child obtains a chronological age equivalent score on a production test of syntax and morphology that would indicate that there is no delay in this linguistic area. However, suppose that on a language sample she evidences semantic word errors and specific problems with spatio-temporal development. The collective results would indicate a specific language disorder related to semantic development. But these results would not be available unless all the available measures (language sample, test scores, and anecdotal records or behavioral observations) were interpreted.

Language delays and language disorders are not mutually exclusive; they may occur simultaneously. For example, the test results of a seven-year-old child may indicate a two-year delay in syntax and morphology, while language sample results suggest specific semantic disorders such as tangentiality and topic closure problems. In this case it is the author's view that the semantic problems should be given priority consideration because intervention in semantics would probably also help the child develop better syntactical and morphological skills.

The interpretation of the test results must be collective. However, it is always possible that using standardized or marketed test results to determine a delay and using the language sample to check for the presence of specific language disorders may result in an interpretation error. The standardized measure makes the assumption that the child is or is not delayed; this assumption must be confirmed by the language sample analysis. In the previous example of the seven-year-old child, the language sample indicated the presence of semantic disorders but did not preclude the fact that there should also have been a noticeable delay in syntax and morphology to support the results of the standardized test. If this delay in syntax and morphology was not indicated in the language sample analysis, then it would mean there's a contradiction in the results. The conclusions from the standardized measures must be confirmed by the language sample analysis; the converse relationship must also be supported.

The interplay among the results obtained from the various measures is similar to hypothesis testing. In hypothesis testing one set of results is used to support or reject another set of results. All contradictions must be resolved through further hypothesis testing and interpretation.

Determining a Language Level

It is possible to determine a language level for those areas of linguistic development that are progressing in an orderly fashion. A general level of language functioning may also be obtained if the child's acquisition of language is delayed in a general, overall way. If a child is language disordered, a statement regarding the child's level of functioning can be misleading and could result in a final error in the diagnostic summary. However, obtaining a language age level or level of language functioning is often a goal of the standardized or marketed test; that is, the final score or test result is reported as a language age equivalence, an age level of functioning, a language age, etc.

Most standardized tests are designed to quantitatively determine a specific child's performance as it relates to other children the *same age*. Since there is an age limitation in the measure, the child who is being assessed must fall within the chronological age level on which the test is normed. Since language is not a good age-related variable beyond the chronological age of seven or eight (except for some semantic skills), most of the content valid standardized measures are not designed for children older than seven or eight.

At this point, a few comments regarding the sample of children used to norm the test are warranted. Most content valid (see Chapter 9) language tests are designed for children between three years of age (beginning of syntax and morphology expansion) and eight years of age (the plateau of basic syntax and morphology development). In general, children between three and eight years of age who reside in the test developer's geographic region are used to develop statistical data for the test items. Stratification procedures (selecting children from various backgrounds and geographic regions) are the best way to randomly choose a sample for establishing normative data. Therefore, even though the sample is assumed to be representative of an entire population, this assumption may be in error as statistically predicted.

Prior to selecting a test for language assessment, the tester should review the characteristics of the original sample population to see if that group's regional characteristics fit the characteristics of the group to be tested. If not, the tester should try out the instrument on some children who are assumed to be without language problems but who fit the racial and cultural background of the children to be tested. The scores of these non-language-delayed children, as a group, should be statistically comparable to the normed group. If the non-language-delayed children do not compare with the norm, the tester has two basic choices: either establish regional norms or do not use the original test data in a normative fashion. Regional norms may also be developed for the children with different racial and cultural backgrounds if the tester wishes to use the test with these children.

When suitable normative data are adapted or developed, then the test results of a specific child may be compared to the norm. Some tests are purported to measure comprehension, while others measure production or imitation.

The content valid language test assesses syntax, morphology, semantics and phonology, or any part of these linguistic areas. Therefore, the results of the test can only be interpreted for the specific areas being assessed. If the test assesses syntax and morphology, then the results for that test pertain only to those two areas of language acquisition.

The organization of the data is usually a product of the test developer's assessment rationale. Some tests are organized to derive a language age or level of ability for a given child as compared to other children. Again, the child's language age for the one test must be reported as it pertains to the area(s) assessed; thus it must not be reported as the child's definitive level of overall language functioning.

Language age is a term suggesting that the child's linguistic skills are comparable to those of a non-language-delayed child of comparable chronological age. Because most school-age children require intervention because of a nonsystematic pattern of acquisition, assessing the child's language abilities in the different linguistic areas is more productive than looking at the language age. An overall level of functioning may be suggestive as part of the final diagnostic summary. For example,

> Sharlene (five years, six months) obtained a score of 58 on the *Test for Auditory Comprehension of Language* (Carrow, 1973), which suggests that her age equivalency for the comprehension of specific syntactical, morphological, and vocabulary skills is three years, six months. The comprehension test results are consistent with a language sample analysis indicating that syntax, morphology, and vocabulary usage are comparable to a three- to four-year-old child.
>
> Examples of Sharlene's best, but typical, utterances include: "Give me that!" "I want milk," "Margie, she my sister, she bought one," "She go upstairs too," "Buy me one?" "What that, please?" "What that do?" "I like read story." During the language sample of 60 consecutive utterances, Sharlene evidenced no semantic language disorders nor problems with language usage or pragmatics. Therefore, Sharlene appears to be using syntax, morphology, and vocabulary of a child three to three years, six months of age, which is about two years below Sharlene's chronological age (five years, six months).

The use of the one norm referenced test coupled with a complete (formal) language analysis (which would have been reported in the main body of the diagnostic report), would be enough to determine whether the child evidences delay or a disorder and what the approximate age level of functioning would be. This assessment, however, would be incomplete as a language diagnostic evaluation. It is important to determine not only the child's problems but also the child's learning strengths in order to make recommendations for remediation.

Language Learning Strengths

Several areas related to the child's language acquisition are important if intervention is to begin after the evaluation. These areas include the processing skills (auditory and visual) and the achievement abilities. (It is assumed that the evaluator always assesses visual and auditory acuity skills, articulation, voice, and fluency behavior.) The processing tests examine the child's intact use of modalities (such as the auditory-to-auditory or the visual-to-auditory circuits) as well as specific skills.

Some of the available tests designed to assess processing include: The Goldman-Fristoe-Woodcock *Battery* (1970, 1974a, 1974b, 1976); *The Illinois Test of Psycholinguistic Abilities* (Kirk, McCarthy, & Kirk, 1968); the *Muma Assessment Program* (Muma & Muma, 1979); and the *Auditory Discrimination Test* (Wepman, 1973). The process information obtained from these tests should substantiate the data obtained from observations and provide additional information concerning specific skills.

Auditory processing problems certainly figure into semantic language disorders since the disruption of language acquisition rests on the development of auditory symbols (aural-oral) to represent visual and auditory information or knowledge. The converse relationship is not true; that is, a child who does poorly on auditory processing tests may not have a semantic language disorder. The purpose of using processing tests is not to determine language disorders but to ascertain the learning strengths. As might be expected, since most of the children with semantic language disorders have auditory processing problems, the majority of these children will evidence strengths in the visual learning skills. However, some children with specific problems (such as with the development of space) may also have visual processing difficulties.

Standardized test results that are reported as a profile of abilities also contribute information regarding the child's learning preferences. For example, a profile interpretation of the *Wechsler Intelligence Scale for Children—Revised* (Wechsler, 1974) will illustrate weaknesses and strengths along areas of learning, because each task may be considered according to its underlying skills. A child who does well on the performance subtests but does poorly on the verbal subtests is obviously learning better from visual and motor experiences than from auditory language experiences. The individual types of items in each subtest may also be analyzed for the processes they require. For example, sequencing story pictures is considered a performance task, but in observing the child's strategies and by asking the child to tell the stories after the section has been administered, the tester can acquire information regarding semantic disorders such as spatio-temporal word errors.

Once the child's learning strengths are determined, the clinician can make decisions regarding language intervention. If visual aids are needed for remediation and intervention, the results of the process tests or profile results should indicate how much visual input is necessary. The need for visual input could range from utilizing an alternate visual mode of communication (e.g., manual communication, Bliss Symbol, or visual reading programs such as Rebus, 1967—for a description of supplemental or alternate modes see Silverman, 1979) to simply positioning the child to receive the speaker's paralinguistic, body, and facial cues.

PURPOSES OF LANGUAGE TESTS

Standardized test results should determine whether the child has a language delay, confirm the presence of specific disorders, provide information regarding the child's language level, and ascertain the child's learning strengths. Integration of the test results for the purpose of developing a diagnostic summary should consider whether the test assessed the process of comprehension, production, and/or imitation. Chapter 1 discussed the assumption parameters of semantic development in relationship to these three processes. The complete language assessment considers each of the three methodologies in order to obtain a comprehensive picture of the child's language abilities.

Comprehension

Most of the widely used language tests developed in the 1970s have been comprehension tests. In this type of test the child is asked to point to a picture representing the word or words that the examiner said. The advantages of this type of testing include:

- The test may be used with a child who has more understanding than the verbal output might suggest.

- The test may be used with shy or reticent speakers to obtain an estimate of what the child's linguistic competence might be.

- The test may be used as a warm-up device since the child does not have to talk to do the task.

Since the pointing responses on the comprehension test are more consistently obtained than some other types of responses, this type of task is easily standardized for responding consistency. Therefore, it is easier to obtain normative data for the comprehension test, as a specific type of task or measure, than for some other productive type of measures.

There are some issues to consider before administering a comprehension measure:

1. The adult's syntactical and morphological stimulus is out of semantic and pragmatic context, which means the child's response is compared to the specific test item and not to the adult's knowledge represented by the stimulus. For example, it is wrong to conclude that a child *knows* "is + verbing" because the child correctly pointed to the representative picture. This conclusion is an overgeneralization of the results. The child responded to the item as did possibly 90 percent of the four year olds used to norm the test.
2. The results of the comprehension test are limited to the child's performance as compared to other children the child's age. A general language level may be obtained only after considering production and language usage skills.
3. The child's ability to respond correctly to comprehension of vocabulary items (as indicated by such stimuli as "point to *girl*" or "point to *climbing*") is restricted by the child's experiences as well as by the semantic limitation of the test item. For example, a child with a semantic language disorder stemming from difficulty associating a lexical tag to an object, action, or event may have extraordinary problems with test items that are line drawings devoid of semantic features. Therefore, the line drawings used for comprehension tasks would be a measure of this child's inability to organize the semantic features, rather than a measure of knowledge about the vocabulary or lexical tag used as the stimulus. Furthermore, the variables of semantic development discussed in Chapter 1 (such as children gradually acquiring referential meaning) must also be considered in interpreting the test results.
4. Even though a comprehension test utilizes a motor response, the directions and stimuli are verbal. This verbal factor can be limiting or problematic for children with auditory language disorders. Since knowledge about the environment may also be learned visually, the auditory stimulus does not assess this other avenue of knowledge. Whenever a comprehension test is administered to a language disordered child, the child's ability to understand the task is an unmeasured variable that may be affecting the overall performance.

Production

Language assessment must include production tests or tasks if the evaluation is to be complete. Recent tests have used a picture format to elicit consistent productions representative of a child's linguistic competence for specific syntactical and morphological constructions (e.g., *Structured Photographic Language Test* by Ellen O'Hara and Janet Dawson Krescheck, 1979). In this kind of test, pictures or photographs are coupled with a verbal stimulus to set a pattern for the child to follow. A pattern or exchange might be:

Adult: The boy is running. (first picture)
Child: The girl is running. (second picture)

The basic assumption underlying the test is that the child understands the pattern and will follow the adult's verbal lead. Children with semantic and pragmatic language disorders may have difficulty following the pattern. For example, an exchange with a language disordered child may proceed as follows:

Adult: The boy is running. (first picture)
Child: This is not a boy. (second picture)

The key to success on the task is setting the directions and patterns so that the child follows with the desired construction.

One problem with this kind of test is that it assumes that if the child produces the portion of the utterance being assessed, then the child is linguistically competent in that type of construction. Therefore, this kind of test does not always give a complete picture of the child's pragmatic and semantic abilities. There are some language disordered children who do well on a pattern task because their basic problem is with the pragmatic aspects of the language, particularly spontaneity and flexibility.

Further research is needed to determine the overall effectiveness of these methodologies for assessing production. The relationship of these test results to spontaneous language sample analyses and comprehension measures also needs to be examined. Until the research provides more answers, it is best to assess production partly by standardized or marketed measures and partly by data from spontaneous language samples. Imitation measures also contribute to the information concerning production skills.

Imitation

The previously cited literature suggests that when a child imitates directly, the imitation does not necessarily reflect comprehension of the meaning and the utterance has little purpose. However, when a child imitates indirectly, then the child integrates the adult's model or stimulus with his or her own level of linguistic competence to produce a structure that is more likely to be representative of the child's true linguistic abilities. The same assumption prevails: The child's production by elicited imitation represents the child's linguistic competence. Even though the pragmatic skills cannot be evaluated by this procedure, the child's actual productions can be analyzed qualitatively for limited semantic skills. However, this procedure cannot explain how these semantic skills are *used* to be communicative. Again, only the qualitative analysis of a spontaneous language sample may determine the range of semantic and pragmatic disorders.

INTEGRATION OF RESULTS

Most individuals who have had some course work or formal training in tests and measurements and who follow test instructions consistently can obtain reliable and valid results on standardized tests. The art of testing and utilizing the test results rests with the examiner's ability to interpret the obtained scores and the corresponding test behaviors. Deciding that the child has a general language disorder and the extent of that problem is accomplished by comparing test results.

Comprehension/Production

In most cases, the child's performance on the comprehension test should be as good as or better than performance on the production test assessing the same syntactical and morphological skills. Exceptions might occur if the productions were automatic, stereotyped, echolalic, or directly imitated. The results of vocabulary tests may or may not be equal to the results of the syntactical and morphological tests because lexical development depends more on the exposure to the word rather than on the acquisition of rules. A child may do better or worse on the vocabulary test depending on the child's experiences as well as on differences between lexical development and syntactical and morphological skills.

Production/Imitation

Spontaneous production and imitation for syntactical and morphological skills should be close to equivalent. However, when the results are not the same, it may suggest that a child who is having difficulty acquiring the essential components of a speech act may imitate at a higher grammatical level than spontaneous productions would suggest.

- This discrepancy in results is produced by the child who expresses specific semantic disorders, general semantic disorders, and pragmatic disorders with or without good comprehension of the input.

- This discrepancy also occurs with the phonological production disorders.

- This discrepancy sometimes occurs when the difference is a delay and is not related to disorders.

The qualitative language sample analysis should confirm or reject these results and then specify the problems.

Determining the Severity

Although many states have developed severity indices in order to provide appropriate and consistent services to all children, there are some general considerations that help determine whether a child's delay or disorder in language warrants remediation or therapeutic intervention:

- If a three-year-old child is not talking (refer to Chapter 2 regarding the social and semantic purpose for language), or if the child is showing other problems in addition to language delay, then a complete diagnostic evaluation is indicated. This evaluation will determine whether or not to begin intervention.

- If a three- to four-year-old child shows a 12-month delay or signs of a disorder, then intervention (based on the child's other developmental behaviors and developmental history) may be indicated. Although the order of language acquisition for most children is relatively invariant for syntax and morphology (see Brown, 1973; Trantham & Pederson, 1976), the rate varies greatly among preschool children.

- If a child between five and eight years of age shows a six- to twelve-month delay and/or signs of disorders with or without other areas of developmental delay, remediation or intervention is probably warranted.

- If a child older than eight has not developed basic syntax and morphology and/or shows signs of language disorders, intervention is most likely warranted.

Although the early years of development are the most variant in normal language acquisition, these early years are probably the most important for effective intervention. Furthermore, the goals and objectives of intervention may change as the child grows and the extent of the limitations becomes more evident. Severity is really the measure of the delay, disorders, and age of the child as well as a comparison of language development to other areas of maturational growth.

WRITING THE RESULTS

In writing the results, the following guidelines should be followed: (1) give the complete names of tests or measures; (2) report the results as the test or measure suggests; (3) interpret the results; (4) integrate the results with the child's chronological age level; and (5) put conclusions into a diagnostic statement or summary. To illustrate these points, the results of three case studies will be considered. The complete report is not presented; only the section that summarizes the language testing is provided.

Case Study 1

Marlene—five years, two months—was referred to the school assessment team (the team included a psychologist, a speech and language clinician, an audiologist, and an education consultant) by her kindergarten teacher, Mr. Randolph. The following results were obtained and written by the speech and language clinician.

> Marlene, a five-year, two-month-old kindergarten student, was referred by her teacher, Mr. Randolph. A language sample of seventy consecutive utterances was obtained from picture stimuli. The first twenty utterances were considered part of the warm-up and were deleted from the quantitative and qualitative analysis. A DSS (Developmental Sentence Score, see Lee, 1974) of 7.07 was derived, which places Marlene's syntactical and morphological development below the 25th percentile for her age and an extrapolation of two years delayed in these areas (5-0 to 5-6). The DSS is consistent with the results of the *Test for Auditory Comprehension of Language* (Carrow, 1973) which suggested that Marlene's comprehension of specific syntactical, morphological, and vocabulary items was two years below her chronological age (5-2). Marlene's raw score was 51 with an age equivalency of 3-2 on the *TACL*.
>
> A qualitative analysis of the language sample utterances revealed the presence of semantic word errors (e.g., *vase* for *cup, table* for *bed, teacher* for *mailman);* neologisms (e.g., *pardot* for *parrot, lamt* for *lamp*—these could be auditory misperceptions; *an eat with* for *fork,* and *Johnny jump* for *jump rope);* space and time errors (e.g., *over* for *next to, runs to* for *runs away, jumps up* for *stands);* syntactic errors related to semantic problems in organization and sequencing (e.g., "The um, girl, um, found, um, the lamp found the girl" and "The teacher, uh, erased, uh the teacher, um erased the teacher").

The specific semantic word errors, syntactic word errors, syntactic-semantic errors, and spatio-temporal word errors suggest that Marlene exhibits specific semantic language disorders with a concomitant language delay of two years in syntax and morphology. Marlene's compliance behavior was consistent with the teacher's report that the child would try to effectively communicate; however, Marlene had difficulties with finishing ideas, with going from one topic to another, and in being referentially clear in spontaneous conversation. Further pragmatic assessment is not warranted until some of the semantic disorders are considered in a remediation program.

As a reminder to the reader, the clinician would also have reported fluency, articulation, and possibly information regarding the structures and functions of the speech mechanism; the psychologist would have reported social and intellectual skills; the audiologist would have reported information regarding hearing; and the education consultant would have reported processing and achievement abilities.

Consistent with the theoretical basis described in the previous chapters, the clinician or teacher would decide to work on the semantic problems directly and/or indirectly through individual or group settings. After reading the test results, the teacher may select those direct tasks (described in Chapter 6 and Chapter 7) aimed at alleviating the semantic disorders.

Since the qualitative and quantitative production skills were consistent with the comprehension results and behavioral observations, further testing, such as by imitation, was not indicated. Furthermore, Marlene was an easy child to test because of her good attending skills and her age and cultural background were appropriate for certain marketed tests. The next child was not so easy to test. Again the speech/language clinician is reporting the results.

Case Study 2

"Mark, a 12-year-old sixth-grade student, was referred for language testing by his resource teacher, Mr. Abrams. Mr. Abrams reported that Mark comes to the resource room for reading and math assistance, two hours a day, each school day of the week."

Mark is beyond the age range in which syntactical and morphological skills are normed on samples of children, so alternative means of using the standardized measures must be considered. Mark is in a regular classroom except for spending two hours daily in a resource situation, which suggests that the use of picture plates designed for younger children would be socially offensive to him. To measure production of syntax and morphology, language sample analyses followed by an imitation procedure such as the *OLSIDI* (Zachman, Husingh,

Jorgansen, & Barrett, 1977), the Menyuk sentence types (Menyuk, 1969), or the *Carrow Elicited Language Inventory* (Carrow, 1974) would be the primary options. Some of the basic comprehension picture plates may be offensive to a 12-year-old child (e.g., *Test for Auditory Comprehension of Language* by Carrow, 1973 or the *Miller-Yoder Test of Grammatical Comprehension, Experimental Edition,* 1972), but tests for "receptive" vocabulary such as the *Peabody Picture Vocabulary Test* (Dunn, 1965), the *Full-Range Picture Vocabulary Test* (Ammons & Ammons, 1948) or the *Boehm Test of Basic Concepts* (Boehm, 1971) may be used either because the material being tested is standardized for the 12-year-old child and/or because the material is developed for administration to individuals older than preschool and primary grade children. The vocabulary tests assess a small portion of semantic development; the other aspects of semantics and pragmatics would have to be assessed by a qualitative language sample analysis.

After the introductory remarks, the following language results section was reported by the clinician:

A language sample was obtained from conversation about school and extracurricular activities. Since Mark did not follow the initial conversation topics, action photographs from the local newspaper office were used to build a conversation around the topics visually represented in the pictures. Forty utterances were obtained from conversation and sixty utterances were obtained from the pictures. The syntax and morphology used in the conversation and in the utterances about the pictures were comparable. Grammatical deviations from adult standard forms included changes in irregular verb usage such as *has came* for *has come* and *aten* for *eaten,* changes in negative forms such as *no* plus *not* and *ain't,* and changes in plural forms such as *mices* for *mice* in the one irregular noun form. These deviations do not affect the communication effectiveness in most situations and considering that Mark showed the ability to use the more advanced grammatical forms (embedding, passive voice, conjoining), his syntax and morphology appear to be adequately developed for communication. This is consistent with Mark's ability to perfectly imitate the grammatical forms on the *Carrow Elicited Language Inventory* (Carrow, 1974). On the *Peabody Picture Vocabulary Test* (Form B), Mark obtained a score of 84, placing him at the 49th percentile for his age, suggesting that receptive vocabulary development is being adequately developed.

[Note that there is no age level for syntax and morphology. To state that Mark had an age level or equivalency of a seven or eight year old in these areas would imply that Mark has a four to five year delay which is an erroneous conclusion. Also observe the fact that a mental age and intelligence quotient were not reported for the *Peabody Picture Vocabulary Test*. The purpose of this evaluation is to determine *vocabulary* abilities; unless mental ages and intelligence quotients are to be interpreted, a job better suited for the psychologist, then the author's personal preference is that these be omitted from the language analysis section.]

A qualitative analysis of the semantic and pragmatic characteristics of the language sample was performed. Results of this analysis indicated the following specific semantic problems: difficulties with referential clarity due to off topic, tangential, and closure problems in addition to some spatio-temporal and specific semantic word errors. Examples of these problems included the following: "Mark, why do you go to the resource room?" Mark responds, "Well, I did my science paper right just one time" (off topic, possibly tangential). "Don't you go to the resource room to get help with your math and reading?" Mark responds, "Did you see the Incredible Hulk?" (off topic). "No, tell me about it." Mark responds, "Well, you see, the Hulk is green, blue like, big monster like man, well uh, he saves women. Well, uh I would like a party, wouldn't you?" (not related to the picture, off topic). "Well, maybe . . . what would we celebrate at the party?" Mark responds, "Perhaps my new bicycle too" (referent is unclear). "We would celebrate about your new bicycle?" Mark responds, "Yes, it's, uh, well it's a shiny new microbike" (semantic word error—maybe recall problem and possibly a semantic neologism). "Is that a minibike?" Mark responds, "Yes, it is, of course" (*of course* is used too often, indicating that it is a filler). "Where do you ride?" Mark responds, "Over rocks, up the streets across the town of course." "Where do you ride across town?" He gives a literal interpretation: "Well, you know, next to, um, right on top of the sidewalks" (definite spatial and temporal problems).

Although Mark has developed adequate syntax, morphology, and phonology, the effectiveness of his language usage is greatly impaired by specific semantic language disorders including problems with off topic and semantic word errors and with spatio-temporal ideas. It is recommended that language remediation for Mark begin with routinization of his environment and with question-answer tasks for alleviating the specific word errors. Spatio-temporal techniques should be used during all activities and should include topic identification (by the addition of visual semantic cues whenever possible), verbal redirection, and the addition of verbal boundaries to his conversation by interruption. These remediation activities may be completed or carried out by the teacher in the classroom, by the resource room teacher, and/or by the language clinician and with the help of the parents.

The previous two reports cited consistent information generated by standardized and language sample measures. Contradictions in test results are quite prevalent and can have a significant effect on the interpretation of results of children with language disorders, since the assumption of systematic and sequential development is violated. In Mark's case, there could have been discussion of the results of the receptive vocabulary test as it relates to the semantic word errors. Although the results are not a contradiction, one might have expected Mark to do poorly with a vocabulary test (one small portion of semantics). Actually, the results support the conclusion that Mark had semantic word errors. Semantic word errors represent an inability to associate an experience with the appropriate lexical tag. Mark was able to learn the tags for specific instances of receptive recall but could not use the tags as they relate to each other and to the environment, a much more generalized language problem. The following case report illustrates the importance of recognizing contradictions and then using this information to tie the diagnostic evaluation together.

Case Study 3

Jerome is a six-year, eleven-month-old second grader referred for a language evaluation by his teacher, Ms. Lincoln, who reported that Jerome "just doesn't make sense sometimes. He's a good child and he's becoming frustrated with classwork and is falling behind the progress of the other children." The school speech and language clinician reported the following information regarding the language assessment.

A language sample of 65 utterances was obtained from picture stimuli and conversation. A language sample analysis of the basic syntactical and morphological structures according to Hannah's (1974) guidelines indicated that Jerome is producing sentence structures comparable to other seven-year-old children, suggesting that syntax and morphology are adequate for his age level. On the *Test for Auditory Comprehension of Language* (Carrow, 1973) Jerome obtained a raw score of 81 with an age equivalency of 5-11. This is not consistent with the syntax and morphology production (at age level in the spontaneous language sample). Since the *TACL* also measures vocabulary, a subtest analysis was performed which indicated that the majority of errors were in isolated vocabulary stimuli (e.g., bicycle). Therefore, the *Peabody Picture Vocabulary Test* (Form A) was administered and Jerome obtained a raw score of 52, which places him at the 13th percentile for receptive vocabulary. This lower-than-age-level performance on the *PPVT* was consistent with the vocabulary subtest of the *TACL*, which had resulted in an age equivalency one year below his chronological age.

A qualitative analysis of the language sample indicated several auditory misperceptions (e.g. *boin* for *join*, but most of these were unintelligible even though articulation was without error on the word test); some semantic word errors related to parts of pictures or meanings of the story rather than to all of the available information (e.g., a chair was described as missing a leg because the boy sitting in the chair obscured the fourth leg, a boy was said to be drowning because he was splashing even though the other pictures related to the story showed the boys playing in the water); and an apparent deficiency in spatio-temporal words and some errors in the terms used (e.g., *on* for *in*, *above* for *in front of*). When Jerome showed signs of anxiety, word finding and verbal perseveration difficulties became evident. Changing the pictures or providing additional semantic cues assisted Jerome's word recall and helped reduce the immediate verbal perseveration. These semantic problems did not negatively affect the pragmatic or overall communicative aspects of his language.

Although some conclusions may be drawn from interpreting the data, further testing of visual and auditory perception, coupled with behavioral observations, is necessary to determine Jerome's learning strengths. Jerome has demonstrated age-level syntax and morphology but has problems in the acquisition, recall, and use of lexicon. Further testing should indicate why these errors exist. Furthermore, the teacher reported that Jerome is missing some of the material in class ("falling behind"). The evaluation to this point has not attempted to explain why Jerome is having difficulty with academic work. Two questions must be considered: (1) Does the specific language problem sufficiently affect the child's learning; and/or (2) Is the language problem secondary to Jerome's overall academic difficulty (possibly related to anxiety, selective attention skills, and/or a different, possibly deprived background of experiences limiting lexicon acquisition)? Perhaps vocabulary deficiency is the main problem; perhaps it is secondary to the learning difficulties. Until there is further assessment of perceptual processing and emotional strength, language results cannot be summarized into a diagnostic statement.

Summary of Assessment

Whenever an older child such as Mark is tested, standardized tests that are not socially offensive to the child may be qualitatively analyzed for error types as compared to adult criteria. This is particularly realistic for imitation tests or for the new production methodologies. With comprehension measures (standardized vocabulary tests and concepts tests such as the *Boehm Test of Basic Concepts* by Boehm, 1971 are exceptions) or indirect verbal comprehension portions of intelligence measures (e.g., sequencing story cards), it is more difficult to justify the qualitative analysis of errors because the assumption of *understanding* changes as the child grows older and passes through stages of meaning and cognitive development. The linguistic competence/performance dichotomy of syntax and morphology appears to plateau and remain relatively constant. Therefore direct or indirect measures of performance may be used with the older child. Although standardized tests in the syntactical and morphological areas do not offer the best means of assessing the older child, the actual skills of the older child or adult may be reported. The standard for assessing competence is not an age of acquisition, as is customary for young children, but a level of ability. The criteria may be obtained from any number of sources reporting sentence types and constructions (e.g., Crystal, 1979; Menyuk, 1969; Trantham & Pederson, 1976).

A language sample analysis that is well documented by examples and sufficiently explained or interpreted according to some specific body of research on normal development expectations will usually be accepted by school districts as a formal measure. This formal measure is further supported by results of standardized tests in related areas. These results help provide a total picture of consistencies or contradictions. Whatever the child's age, communication skills must be considered even if the child's performance is considered prelinguistic.

There are some principles that may be used as guidelines to total language assessment:

1. Pick a content valid instrument and be sure that the normative data, if used, are suitable for the child being tested.
2. If the child's language production is generally less than three or four lexical terms per utterance, then consider the following in assessing the young child or the child with low language level:
   a. Is the child's behavioral responsiveness to the environment consistent with the child's level of production?
   b. What does the child respond to and how does the child respond?
   c. What is the child's mean length of utterance (see Brown, 1973)?
   d. What are the child's prelinguistic skills (see McLean & Snyder-McLean, 1978)?
   e. If the child has a chronological age between three and eight years (approximately), what is the child's performance on comprehension and imitation measures of syntax and morphological development?
   f. How do syntax and morphology on the standardized measures compare to the language sample analysis?

   g. What are the results of the qualitative language sample analysis (see Chapter 4)?
   h. What are the child's learning preferences?
   i. What types of communication is the child capable of doing—for example, does the child read?
3. If the child's language production is generally greater than three or four lexical terms per utterance, then include the following in the assessment:
   a. If a quantitative measure of syntax and morphology is used, does it match with the comprehension measure of the same skills? For an overview of available language measures, consult the material in diagnostic sections of texts (e.g., Darley, 1979; Darley & Spriestersbach, 1978; Nation & Aram, 1977; McLean & Snyder-McLean, 1978).
   b. What processes or strategies does the child employ? (This is obtained either through tests and/or through observation.)
   c. What are the results of the qualitative analysis of the child's language sample (see Chapter 4)?
   d. What are the consistencies and contradictions in the informal and standardized test results?
   e. How do the results compare to the referral complaint, to the behavioral observations, and to the academic or task performance?
4. Relate the test results to comparable criteria of other test results. In other words, results of a test that measures syntax and morphology should be consistent with other measures that either overlap or are very similar to the linguistic skills being assessed.
5. Interpret the findings of the test results according to knowledge about normal and disrupted language comprehension, production, and acquisition.
6. Compare the results to test norms, criteria, and to other tests when preparing the diagnostic summary statement and recommendations.

Questions

1. What types of questions are answered by standardized tests?
2. What types of language measures are used with children older than eight?
3. Why are the basic assumptions that underlie assessment of a language level or age younger than 3.0 different from the assumptions that underlie assessment of a language level or age greater than 3.0?
4. What assumptions underlie tests for linguistic competence in syntax and morphology?
5. Why must both comprehension and production be assessed?

REFERENCES

Ammons, R. B., & Ammons, H. S. *Full-range picture vocabulary test*. Missoula, Mt.: Psychological Test Specialists, 1948.

Boehm, A. E. *Boehm test of basic concepts*. New York: Psychological Corporation, 1971.

Brown, R. *A first language: The early stages*. Cambridge, Mass.: Harvard University Press, 1973.

Carrow, E. *Test for auditory comprehension of language*. Boston, Mass.: Teaching Resources Corporation, 1973.

Carrow, E. *Carrow elicited language inventory*. Boston, Mass.: Teaching Resources Corporation, 1974.

Crystal, D. *Working with LARSP*. New York: Elsevier North Holland, 1979.

Darley, F. L. (Ed.). *Evaluation of appraisal techniques in speech and language pathology*. Reading, Mass.: Addison-Wesley Publishing Corp., 1979.

Darley, F. L., & Spriestersbach, D. C. *Diagnostic methods in speech pathology*. New York: Harper & Row, 1978.

Dunn, L. M. *Peabody picture vocabulary test*. Circle Pines, Minn.: American Guidance Services, 1965.

Goldman, R., Fristoe, M., & Woodcock, R. W. *Battery of auditory tests* including *GFW auditory selective attention tests*, 1976; *GFW auditory memory tests*, 1974; *GFW sound-symbol*, 1974; and *GFW test of auditory discrimination*, 1970. Circle Pines, Minn.: American Guidance Service, Inc.

Hannah, E. P. *Applied linguistic analysis*. Northridge, Ca.: Joyce Motion Picture Co., 1974.

Kirk, S. A., McCarthy, J. J., & Kirk, W. D. *The Illinois test of psycholinguistic abilities (Rev. ed.)*. Urbana, Ill.: University of Illinois, 1968.

Lee, L. L. *Developmental sentence analysis*. Evanston, Ill.: Northwestern University Press, 1974.

McLean, J., & Snyder-McLean, R. *A transactional approach to early language training*. Columbus, Ohio: Charles E. Merrill, 1978.

Menyuk, P. *Sentences children use*. Cambridge, Mass.: MIT Press, 1969.

Miller, J., & Yoder, D. *Miller-Yoder test of grammatical comprehension, experimental edition*. Madison, Wis.: University of Wisconsin Bookstore, 1972.

Muma, J. R., & Muma, D. B. *Muma assessment program*. Lubbock, Tex.: Natural Child Pub., 1979.

Nation, J. E., & Aram, D. M. *Diagnosis of speech and language disorders*. St. Louis, Mo.: C.V. Mosby Co., 1977.

O'Hara, E., & Krescheck, J. D. *Structured photographic language test*. Sandwich, Ill.: Janelle Publishing Co., 1979.

Rebus Materials. Salt Lake City, Utah: Word Making Productions, 1973. Peabody Rebus Reading Program. R.W. Woodcock. Circle Pines, Minn.: American Guidance Services, 1967.

Silverman, F. *Communication for the speechless*. New York: Prentice-Hall, 1979.

Trantham, C. R., & Pederson, J. K. *Normal language development*. Baltimore, Md.: Williams & Wilkins Co., 1976.

Wechsler, D. *Manual for the Wechsler intelligence scale for children—revised*. New York: Psychological Corporation, 1974.

Wepman, J. M. *Auditory discrimination test (Rev. ed.)*. Chicago, Ill.: Language Research Associates, 1973.

Zachman, L., Husingh, R., Jorgansen, C., & Barrett, M. *The oral language sentence imitation diagnostic (or screening) inventory* (OLSIDI or OLSISI). Moline, Ill.: Lingui Systems, 1977.

CHAPTER OBJECTIVES

- write the goals for a child with spatio-temporal difficulties.

- write the objectives for a child with spatio-temporal problems.

- list techniques to remediate space and time problems.

- design appropriate activities for facilitating space and time development.

- develop a remediation program for a child with space and time problems based on input from a qualitative analysis of a language sample coupled with behavioral observations and standardized test results.

- explain the difference between intervention for vocabulary building and intervention for facilitation of conceptual knowledge.

- describe compensatory skills that may develop in a child who has space, time, or quantity problems.

- describe behaviors that may suggest a language problem of space and time.

- explain why it is sometimes said that all language delayed and/or language disordered children will eventually evidence problems in space and time.

- describe the range of space and time problems for different kinds of children.

Chapter 6

Remediation Activities and Techniques for Spatio-Temporal Disorders

The world was up but I was down, at best There couldn't be an in-between and I couldn't go forward because there wasn't a backward And my future didn't exist because I couldn't find "next," "after," or "later" . . . until, I realized today was me and yesterday was backward and tomorrow would be better!

This chapter is devoted to the specific characteristics of children with space and time disorders and their concomitant remediation procedures. Children who experience difficulty with space and time development often exhibit behavioral characteristics or symptoms that are confused with other disorders. Consequently, the other problems are treated but the child remains a frustrating challenge to the teacher, parent, and remediation specialists. This chapter will provide an in-depth discussion of the space-time language disorder briefly characterized in Chapter 3, including the associated behavioral characteristics, the historical perspective to remediation, and the present intervention techniques and activities.

Remediation techniques for use in home, clinical, and/or class settings will be described. Examples of lesson plan goals, objectives, and criteria for progressing to the next level of difficulty, as well as basic procedures for taking data are included. Further discussion on data taking will be found in Chapter 9.

SPATIO-TEMPORAL CONCEPTS

The period of time between infancy and first grade is critical to the development of spatio-temporal concepts. During these first few years, the essential perceptual characteristics of the planes of space are integrated and attached to the society's use of specific lexicon. Only when the child has become accustomed to the spatial organization of the immediate environment (usually by first grade), does time lexicon denoting nonsimultaneous events (for example, "next," "before," "after," etc.) begin to emerge consistently. By the time most children are eight years of age, the basic space and time concepts are ingrained into daily living. This gradual process, although still very theoretical in nature, is presumptive, expedient (considering the complexity of what is being learned), and effective.

When the normal acquisition is slowed down, interrupted, distorted, or incomplete, the child exhibits several characteristics of a language disorder that affects academic skills. Figure 6-1 is a schematic representation of the points of possible breakdown in the acquisition of spatio-temporal concepts: sensory input integrative of sensory information, perceptual integration, attachment of lexical markers, and/or production.

This same schema could also apply to any semantic concept which, as suggested in Chapter 1, could include all referents, propositions, predications, and

---

Figure 6-1 Disruption Sites for Space and Time Concepts

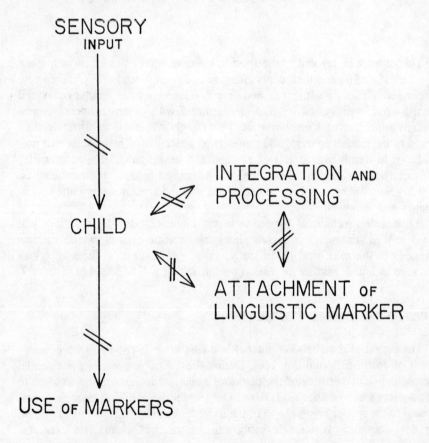

modulations of the language. Since spatio-temporal concepts permeate the hierarchical progression of language, a child may experience difficulty anywhere along the continuum of development. Much can be learned about the acquisition of these concepts by viewing the resultant disorders.

Spatio-temporal problems eventually occur in any child with a language delay and/or language disorder. To illustrate this latter point, language corpora from children diagnosed as mentally retarded, learning disabled, language delayed, and emotionally disturbed will be analyzed independently to isolate problems with space and time concepts. The purpose of illustrating the range of children affected is to demonstrate the importance of dealing with these difficulties.

Mentally Retarded Children

In most mentally retarded children, the syntax and morphology milestones of the first few years emerge slower than expected; language development, however, emerges systematically (e.g., Kahn, 1975; Lackner, 1968; Lenneberg, Nichols, & Rosenberger, 1969; Miller & Yoder, 1974; Morehead & Ingram, 1973). By the time the mentally retarded child is six to eight years of age or older, the language development appears to show other problems associated with semantic development. The severity of these problems seems to be related to the gap between production of syntax and morphology and the underlying semantic basis, rather than to the child's overall general level of language acquisition (Schauer, 1978). Although further research is needed to support this hypothesis, it seems that the semantic area of language depends on early experiences for normal development. It may be that the mentally retarded child does not approach these early experiences in the same manner as the normal child. Whatever the difference, the semantic problems are apparent.

Structural forms may be learned or taught. However, as long as the semantic basis is weak, space and time concepts, not to mention qualifiers and quantifiers, will be problematic. Of course, these concepts are directly connected to cognitive abilities. The language system is also positively affected by the development of additional language and more complex cognitive abilities. The weak semantic basis may possibly be a result of slower learning, or it may be that the mentally retarded child is facing a latency plateau in learning. The effects of this plateau are seen in the older mentally retarded child. Thus by the time some mentally retarded children acquire enough language to deal with these concepts, they are adolescents and are involved in educational programs that stress vocational training and improved intelligibility for job placement rather than language development. It is also a possibility that intervention programs for the retarded do not facilitate enough of the semantic basis. In that case, the space and time problems are inevitable. By the time enough language has been developed to begin expressing space and time concepts, intervention may have disrupted the sequential and systematic acquisition so that the child exhibits a disorder.

The following examples were obtained from a study (Schauer, 1978) that examined two groups of children's language matched individually and by group according to mental age from standardized psychological tests used for special education placement. Children in Group A were considered educably retarded, with a chronological age of approximately 7.0 and a mental age of 5.0. Children in Group B had a chronological age and mental age of 5.0. The purpose of the study was to determine the similarities or differences in language between these groups when language was analyzed for syntax, morphology, and semantics. The children in each group were asked to talk about the same pictures after receiving formalized instructions about the task. The sampler responded to the children's responses with nondirective comments such as "oh," "uh, huh," "I see," etc.

The results of the study indicated that both groups of children developed syntax and morphology (determined by Hannah's Applied Linguistic Analysis and Developmental Sentence Scores) that were equivalent to a corresponding mental age. However, the two groups of children differed in the number of semantic errors (Hannah, 1974). The following segment is presented to illustrate the types of semantic problems associated with space and time that were found with the retarded children but not found with the "normal" group of children when a qualitative analysis was applied.

Retarded—Group A	*Normal—Group B*
Picture 1	*Picture 1*
This boys got his clothes.	The clothes are too big.
He was asleep.	One sleeve is too long.
He waked up.	I can't even see one arm.
He ate breakfast.	
Picture 2	*Picture 2*
This boy, he getting his shirt on.	One of the buttons fell off, I think.
He's biting his shirt so he can go outside.	The shirt's too small for him.
Picture 3	*Picture 3*
He's putting ice in the shirt.	What's the boy doing? He's sticking the ice down her shirt.

The boy in the first picture realizes that he is wearing the wrong size shirt; it is definitely too big. Notice that the retarded children (Group A) ignored the relevant perceptual features related to size. In the second picture, the boy has put on a shirt that is too small and he's looking at the buttons trying to pull it together to get the shirt fastened. Notice the one semantically bizarre example from Group A: the child thought that the boy in the picture was biting his shirt because he wanted to go outside. For Picture 2, none of the retarded subjects mentioned that the shirt didn't fit. Again the perceptual attributes for the picture were ignored, possibly not acquired, and/or suggestive of different learning preferences. The only unusual semantic intent expressed by Group B was the belief that maybe the boy was looking at his shirt because he lost a button. This was a reasonable alternate explanation of the picture.

In the third picture, a boy is putting something cold down a girl's shirt. The normal subjects attended to the perceptual detail and appropriately marked their utterances with the correct prepositions of space. The retarded children did not. The retarded children (Group A) used "in" for "on," did not recognize the semantic relationship between the child receiving the ice and the one putting it down the shirt, etc. These are just a few examples from the study to illustrate that even when the syntax and morphology are developing sequentially and according to what might be expected of a child with a corresponding mental age, the retarded child still has problems putting semantic relationships together and marking them linguistically with the appropriate spatio-temporal markers.

Language Delayed and Language Disordered Children

Children who develop their language skills slower than other children do not evidence problems with space and time unless the delay persists into or beyond the five- to seven-year-old period. Every delayed child five years or older that the author has seen is beginning to experience difficulty with space and time concepts. This suggests that most school-age children who are in language remediation programs are probably language disordered. The major exception to the disorder pervasiveness is the group of children who are second language learners, including those that might be dialectically different.

The fact that older language delayed children begin to evidence difficulty in acquiring space and time concepts, aside from the natural systematic and sequential order of other language skills is not unexpected. Space development is related to experiences corresponding to knowledge, perceptual processing intactness, and self-concept development (three areas often listed problematic for language delayed children). Time follows the progress of space development. Temporal concepts are expressed by verb complex modulations and the acquisition of time vocabulary. Since language delayed children have trouble with verb complexity, perhaps the time element to verbing is partially semantic in nature and a product of the time problem.

The child with a general language disorder will evidence spatio-temporal difficulties because at least one of the processes prior to or at the output level is being negatively affected. Children may show a specific language disorder

(Chapter 3) without semantic word errors related to space and time. And, conversely, some children's language output may be incomprehensible because of space and time difficulties. The following segment of language is from a child who is chronologically five years, six months and language delayed syntactically and morphologically by two years according to standardized measures of imitation and comprehension. The problems with general space, time, and referential concepts are beginning to emerge.

> "Put the little doll here."
> "Now, he sitting on box." (in the box.)
> "See!"
> "The man, he big?" (The referent to big is unclear—all of the dolls were the same size. Maybe "big" referred to men being big in contrast to the size of most boys.)
> "Here he goed too." (The action is present progressive as the child is making the boy go as the utterance is made.)
> "Come on, Ms. Smith, come on!"
> "Make the man go too."
> "What's this?" (It's a refrigerator—it goes in the kitchen.)
> "Me go right here." (Where are you?)
> "Here, see?" (What room are you in?)
> "Here come the mama!" (Jimmy, listen! Is this the bedroom?)
> "No." (What is the name of this room?)
> "Fidgator' room!"

From this language segment, it is easy to see that this child has difficulties with understanding semantic relationships of place and/or understanding the child's own relationship to places. The problems of space and time are evident. Also notice the increased use of introducers ("this," "here"), labels, and indefinite referents ("This man," "no name," etc.)—typical of children with semantic word errors. It should be restated that problems with space and time are actually a type of semantic word error, with quantifiers and qualifiers also being affected.

Emotionally Disturbed Children

The emotionally disturbed child may have difficulty relating to the here and the now, but this child's language evidences a psychological disorganization, not usually a spatio-temporal semantic word disorder, even though some of the same characteristics are observed in the language. These children need many of the same organizational properties of remediation suggested later in the chapter, but they do not need direct intervention aimed at teaching space and time concepts. The language problem of the emotionally disturbed child is related more to the linguistic product or pragmatic skills than to the content or semantic skills.

An example of language produced by an emotionally disturbed nine-year-old male illustrates the problems with reality associated with what appears to be spatial and temporal confusion. The types of language difficulties evidenced also depend on the child's specific emotional problems. This child had been diagnosed as schizophrenic by the American Psychiatric Association classifications.

1. "My mother drowned my dog this morning."
   "She did? Are you sure?"
2. "Yeh. She went to the creek and held its head in the water until it was dead."
   "What was your dog's name?"
3. "Well, his name is Charlie and he's a cocker spaniel."
   "Where does he live?"
4. "Well, my mother drowned him in the creek this morning."
   "I'm sorry to hear that. Was it an accident?"
5. "She fell in on top of Charlie and held his head down in the water."
   "Where is your dog now?"
6. "Well, he's in the house asleep by the fire in the kitchen."

The child did have a dog, but the dog had not drowned nor had he ever lost a dog. This same story was repeated every few days. Although the child appears to be temporally confused, the disorganization is more in terms of the child's approach to pragmatic skills. Children who are emotionally disturbed often utter propositional content that does not represent what the child intends. Instead of wanting to talk about the dog, this child may have wanted help with his homework. The inability to express one's intent (that is, to use the appropriate illocutionary force indicating devices described in the essential rule component) results in content confusion on the part of the hearer. In most situations, the hearer responds to the child's "dog story" and not to the underlying intent. The child's anxiety is perpetuated because the needs are not met and the hearer's frustration also increases. Most of these problems are better approached from the standpoint of the pragmatic remediation techniques suggested in Chapter 8.

Learning Disabled Children

This type of child is discussed last because most children who have no significant problems except for a spatio-temporal language disorder would most likely be found in resource facilities or programs for the learning disabled. Many of the remedial or reading readiness programs use the same types of activities suggested in this chapter for use with children who exhibit space and time learning difficulties. Once these children are in a remedial program aimed directly at the language skills, prognosis is excellent for quick and effective gains.

BEHAVIORAL CHARACTERISTICS

Children with specific spatio-temporal difficulties have a basic semantic problem in acquiring or assigning perceptual attributes to denote spatial dimensions and/or time. On the surface, the problem is evidenced by a disorganization in the linguistic flow from one proposition to another proposition. For example, "My dog is black" and "My dog is at home" are two separate ideas joined in thought by position and simultaneous time—and, in this case, not by linguistic skill. To join these ideas linguistically—"My black dog is at home"—requires the linguistic embedding of one idea into another. The enjoining or conjoining of ideas, no matter at what level of linguistic ability, is difficult for these children. The difficulty may not be with the linguistic skills but with the combination of thoughts or the temporal sequence of events required in conjoining and embedding.

The child's disorganization affects daily activities, including: (1) following directions; (2) completing assignments; (3) explaining events; (4) reading by auditory skills, which requires sound blending in sequence; (5) performing advanced math; and (6) learning new activities such as games. The child's lack of organization becomes more noticeable as the occasional "spaced out" appearance becomes more of the child's personality. Teachers become frustrated with the child who forgets to come back at the appropriate time after lunch or who consistently passes the wastebasket without throwing away the milk carton. As more language skills are acquired, the internal confusion regarding spatial orientation and temporal organization results in other language problems. These problems include: (1) incessant verbalization (lack of topic closure because the child doesn't appear to know when the right amount of information has been given to affect a hearer in an intended manner); (2) reverbalization or vocal reiteration of material as a self-help or self-organizing device that can be audibly disruptive to hearers; and (3) off target or off topic utterances. The "funny" sayings or comments become more obvious as the academic difficulties increase.

Basic comprehension or achievement tests may show the child doing well up to second grade (about seven to eight years of age). At this point the child begins to lose ground when compared to other children the same age, because the sequencing of events by time becomes more of an academic factor. Sometimes a perceptual problem in vision and/or hearing is diagnosed. Remediation in these areas aids academic learning but may not help the child to organize the environment linguistically. The child, who appears to be not quite aware of what is happening in the classroom or on the playground, is often referred to the psychologist. Although the psychologist may help the child deal with feelings of failure and confusion, the language disorder may persist.

There is some indication that if no other problem exists, these children will develop adaptive behaviors and/or catch up with their age group. Nevertheless, the risk of academic failures and the detrimental effects of these failures on self-concept necessitates early intervention. Furthermore, there are adults and adolescents who have not acquired adaptive behavior, and those who do acquire adaptive skills often have a language disorder that is limiting.

The following case studies illustrate how spatio-temporal difficulties can interrupt language acquisition. A range of severity is represented.

Case 1

David, an active six year old, was described by his teacher as follows: "He just isn't socially mature enough to pass into the first grade. His work is satisfactory but he doesn't always get it in on time. David follows the other children and is quite serious. When we have share time, David just doesn't always make sense. He has all of the ideas but the words just don't go together."

David had the following conversation with an adult:

> *Adult:* "So you saw the fireworks."
> *David:* "Yes, I saw the fireworks at the Ohio stadium."
> *Adult:* "Oh, you went to the stadium."
> *David:* "Yes, we saw the fireworks on TV."
> *Adult:* "You saw the fireworks on TV?"
> *David:* "We went to the stadium yesterday."
> *Adult:* "Yesterday? But the fireworks were Saturday and yesterday was Monday. Did you see the fireworks at the stadium?"
> *David:* "My Dad watched them on TV."
> *Adult:* "Your dad saw the fireworks on TV and you saw the fireworks at the stadium?"
> *David:* "My dad works, usually, and this morning he flew the plane."

The adult never did find out if this child saw fireworks at the stadium, on TV, or both. David was also the boy who believed that elevators did not move, but the buildings did; and that if a picture of an airplane was held above his head, the plane was taking off. If the picture of the plane was held on the ground, the plane was landing. Relatives had encouraged the parents to bring David to a speech clinic because they believed that David just didn't "sound right."

From the language segment, it is evident that David cannot answer questions that require a space or time referent. It is also difficult for him to sequence a story or follow an idea from the previous speaker's utterance. Due to David's age and lack of academic failure, the people in his environment perceive his difficulties as "sounding funny," a layman's interpretation of a mild problem, at this time.

Case 2

Danny, an eight-year-old second grader, did well in the first grade but dislikes second grade because of increasing academic failure. Danny's parents are concerned about his learning and most of all about his newly acquired negative attitude about school. It was reported that Danny could not follow the longer directions given in second grade, that sight reading was quickly accomplished but that the learning of auditory sequencing skills for advanced reading was almost impossible, that story problems in math were difficult, and that even socialization had new complications. Because Danny couldn't memorize required Bible lessons—even though he understood the lessons and could repeat them in everyday language—and because he couldn't learn new games without watching, other children in the parochial school teased him. Music lessons were more difficult with second-grade music books that didn't have the visual keys; trying to retell an event or story was a disastrous and frustrating experience. However, Danny's language was quite good for very structured tasks in which the referents were limited. Occasionally, he would try to figure out the appropriate prepositions or spatial relations. For example, "The man is in the garage . . . no, he is through the garage." One conversation, his most difficult language task, was recorded as follows:

> Adult: "What did you do at school today?"
> Danny: "Played and worked and ate lunch."
> Adult: "What did you do after lunch."
> Danny: "Oh, we went home?"
> Adult: "I mean, right after lunch . . . as soon as you finished eating."
> Danny: "Oh! We had recess and I had to do my math since the grade was not so good this time it was better. I didn't write the numbers, you know, just right, and so I had recess yesterday. Oh, maybe today, too."

Adult: "You didn't do well on your math."

Danny: "Oh! Yes, this time I did the numbers just like, you know, well, I just can't remember, you know . . . well, I just don't know what else to say."

From this conversation, it is apparent that Danny cannot sequence or associate events by temporal lexicon. Furthermore, he can't respond to the questions of nonspecific time, such as "What did you do after . . . ?" The child can't even answer (with the necessary referential meaning) the question about the present. The fact that Danny is old enough to experience academic failure and to recognize his abilities is evident when he says, "I just don't know what else to say."

Case 3

The following seventeen-year-old Down's Syndrome adolescent is describing the party from which she has just returned:

1. "I had about two cookies at the party, that's it."
   "Are you still on your diet?"
2. "Yeah, I'm still on it but I just had two."
   "That's all."
3. "Well, I bought about three cookies."
   "Oh."
4. "I ate two and that's all I ate."
   "Uh, huh."
5. "I bought one for my boyfriend."
   "You did?"
6. "There's a cookie in my pocket and stuff."
7. "I'll give that to him."
8. "And then as soon as he comes back, I'll give it to him."
9. "He might come back around a little later."
   "What for?"
10. "Well, he might go down to see his friends."
11. "I was just hangin' around down on second."
    "Was the party yesterday?"
12. "No, it's today."
13. "Down here in the chapel." (Note: The chapel is outside the building.)
    "What are they doing?"

14. "They were singing Halloween songs and part of Christmas songs."
15. "And as soon as they got done singing trick-or-treat songs."
16. "So they're all done trick-or-treat songs."
17. "So they stopped singin' and we all clapped."
18. "After we clapped, we all sat on the floor."
19. "Then I sang a song, too."
20. "So all of us they said come and get it."
21. "They lined the cookies up on the table there."
22. "And so we have a few cookies."
23. "I had two and I ate two and that's all I ate."
24. "And I bought one more makes three."
25. "Then I can give one to John."
26. "So he can have one to eat."
27. "If he comes back I'll give it to him."
28. "And that's all I did."

This adolescent had made significant progress in a language therapy program aimed at facilitating the semantic concepts. Prior to that program, she had been in a program for increasing syntax and morphology, and she was quite impressive at drill tasks for structures as well as for imitation. Prior to the semantic concept approach, her spontaneous language was limited to responses of four to five words at maximum. She once allowed a washing machine to overflow and as she watched it, she was asked, "Why?" Her answer implied that no one expected the initiation of language or the performance of a speech act. Again, the semantic basis that is developed for use greatly affects overall language development. Even though this client had made significant progress, it is apparent that she still has some space and time problems related primarily to performing a speech event or a series of propositions. Her use of certain time lexicon and verb markers is indicative of the area of weakness.

In the three previous language samples, it should be noted that the clarity of the message was greatly hindered by the lack of referential specificity with regard to space and particularly with regard to sequencing time between two events. Other examples of spatio-temporal disorders were provided in Chapters 3 and 4.

Before beginning the next section on remediation, the main principle about space and time may be stated: *A child's life is organized by how the objects, actions, and events are related. The words describing these perceived relationships are spatial and temporal in nature. Unless these relationships are easily and readily expressible, an auditory form of communication may be perplexing. Undo the perplexity and the child's world becomes organized.*

REMEDIATION

Language clinicians and educators have for many years recognized the need to teach spatio-temporal concepts to language delayed and disordered children. The techniques for facilitating space and time have often promoted labels but no concepts. For example, in some programs a child was given a comprehension test in which the child was to point to an object or picture depicting "in the box" as opposed to "on" and "under" the box. If the child pointed correctly, then the adult interpreted the response as *knowing the concept*.

Unfortunately, space and time concepts are gradually acquired, and it's quite possible for the child to respond correctly and consistently in one context but not in another context. The same child who knew "in the box" might say that the "chicken is on the dirt" or "on the garden." Standardized tasks that ask the child to point to and/or put something in relationship to another object explain how the child does on these tasks compared to other children the same age. If these tasks are used in training, they indicate how well the child learns that particular task but not necessarily if the child knows a concept.

REMEDIATION PROCEDURES

There are several critical factors to consider when devising remediation programs to facilitate or teach space and time concepts:

- Production of the vocabulary terms in one context doesn't indicate that the child has mastered the dictionary-like definition that an adult might possess. Dictionary usages should not be expected of children younger than 12 years of age.
- The use of these spatio-temporal concepts, appropriate or judged to be inappropriate by adult standards, assist a child in learning all of the possible meanings.
- Recent literature, referenced in Chapter 1, regarding vocabulary growth should be considered prior to choosing the contexts for facilitating the concepts.
- The greater the variety of settings and usages used for teaching, the more likely the concept will be learned.

Each of these factors will be considered in the approach outlined for dealing with space and time problems.

The following language segment was collected from a child who struggled with spatio-temporal concepts. The segment will be analyzed qualitatively and then the techniques will be explained. The examiner asks, "Did you like baseball?"

"I didn't, I didn't like hitting, once, for a few times, like in the last game I hit, hit a first base but ended up going to second base, I ended up going to two bases and, and ended going to first base for the pitcher had already, uh, well, already whoever threw the ball hit— ended up getting to third base, and, the first base cuz at least I already was on the base he wanted, so he went out and I went to second base (pause) to get the ball."

This child had enough visual-motor coordination to play baseball as well as other children his age. But according to this short, but typical, segment the child's linguistic expression about baseball is less than adequate for a ten year old. The child's attachment of the lexicon to the activity is less than satisfactory. The teacher reported that in the classroom this child didn't follow directions well and didn't finish his work. He wasn't learning how to read beyond sight vocabulary nor was he learning advanced math skills.

Results from a qualitative language sample analysis, coupled with information from the classroom and results from standardized tests, indicate that the problem is with the acquisition of space and time concepts.

Johnny begins to answer the question, "Did you like baseball?" with the utterance, "I didn't, I didn't like hitting, once, for a few times . . . ." There are two unclear messages: (1) Did he like everything about baseball except hitting, or (2) Did he not like hitting one specific time or times? Notice that these messages are ambiguated by the redundancy within the temporal segment "for a few times." Most speakers would say *"once in a while"* or *"sometimes"* or *"occasionally,"* etc. Johnny attempts to clarify the idea that he didn't like hitting sometimes by giving an example: "Like in the last game I hit, hit a first base but ended up going to second base, I ended up going to two bases." In the latter part of the utterance, the hearer is not sure if Johnny made a double play or if Johnny ran to second base on another play that wasn't mentioned. The timing of the events is not clear and is further confused by Johnny continuing the story: " . . . and, and ended going to first base for the pitcher had already, uh, well already, whoever threw the ball hits." Now, Johnny is back on first base. The time sequence is further ambiguated: the hearer wonders if this is the same play or Johnny's next turn at bat.

Johnny's story needed some temporal markers tied between specific referents to give the relationship among events. He tries to explain who the pitcher is so that the hitter and pitcher are not confused, but he ambiguates the utterance by not using specific referents: *"Whoever* threw the ball, hits." The relationship between actions is also confused "I hit a first base," resulting in syntactical errors and semantic confusion on the part of the hearer.

Johnny is similar to many children with spatio-temporal problems, because he realizes he isn't very effective at explaining the event. This recognition may stem from his own realization of his errors and/or from the nonverbal feedback of the hearer who is showing signs of bewilderment. When Johnny realizes that the story is not flowing very well, he tries to explain by saying, " . . . ended up getting to third base, and, and first base." If the reader has been keeping track, Johnny has been to first, second, first, third, and back to first base with no indication of the time at which these actions took place. Johnny gives a reason for going to the last first base in the series: " . . . cuz at least I already was on the base he wanted." This latter statement shows time redundancy errors ("at least" and "already") and again the same problem with connecting semantic relationships.

Johnny's use of indefinite or referential words without an antecedent is also problematic. For example, the pronoun "he" in the last utterance of Johnny's story can only refer to the pitcher, but pitchers are not usually "wanting" bases, " . . . so he went out and I went to second base (pause) to get the ball." Most baseball fans realize that if a player is running the bases, that player isn't also trying to get the ball. The ambiguous explanation could be clarified with a few correctly placed time and space markers:

> "Sometimes I didn't like hitting—like in the last game. I hit the ball and ran to first and then on to second. Then my friend hit a ball, and I couldn't go to third because the ball was thrown there, so I ran back to second; but the guy on first was already coming. So he was tagged out and I stayed on second base."

Notice that vocabulary specifying the objects, actions, and events is also needed in the revised paragraph. The need for referents is not uncommon with spatio-temporal problems. The child has difficulty organizing the requisite perceptual and functional attributes into vocabulary concepts—whether of space, time, or other quantifiers or qualifiers. Therefore, teaching any of these concepts as vocabulary words will not help the child organize the environment. The child needs organization through the concepts, not through the linguistic tags.

Routinization in Remediation

The first step in remediation is to use language to organize as much of the child's environment as possible. This means that the child needs to know what is going to happen, where it will happen and when it will happen. The child needs this kind of information for the home environment as well as for the school setting. The information should be given consistently and clearly by the same people and at the same time of the day for the same activities. For example:

"Billy, it's Monday and you need to get ready for school. Then we'll have breakfast. After breakfast, I'll take you to school. After school is over, I want you to pick up your room before Dad comes home for dinner. Your sister is helping with dinner tonight, so you will be expected to help with the dishes. After the dishes are done, we'll work on your homework, watch a little TV, get ready for bed, and then go to bed."

These delineations of events must be carried out as told to the child.

The same verbal organization should also be provided at school. Children without a good grasp of spatio-temporal concepts will follow others' action, but the dependency creates problems when the child is expected to work independently and finish work within a certain time frame. Even when a child can recognize numbers on a clock, the child doesn't always have the internal clock.

There are a few children who learn to adjust and adapt by developing compensatory skills. For example, a 29-year-old female employed in a sheltered workshop was referred for a language evaluation. This individual had been diagnosed as trainable retarded, but the social worker questioned this diagnosis. The client was married and quite self-sufficient. When she was a child her family had allowed her to stay home from school. She explained this as follows: "Well, I was sort of special. My mama let me stay home to help her cook and all." When asked why she didn't go to school with her brothers and sisters, she said, "Well, I did go to school for a time—maybe third, fourth grade, I don't know. But the school said I was stupid and couldn't learn to read and write, but mom said I wasn't so she just didn't ready me for school. I stayed home and helped."

This client's eight brothers and sisters received some form of vocational and/ or professional training beyond high school. The client had developed outstanding compensatory skills to make up for being unable to auditorily match visual symbols and thus being able to learn to read, write, tell time, learn the names of numbers, and denote space, time, or quantity. She had taught herself many skills, including calling taxis or doctors by matching the picture or number on the appointment card with the number in the yellow pages; being able to call her family and friends by visually matching memorized phone numbers to the phone digits; picking up her seven-year-old child at school or getting her ready for an appointment or for school and never being late. When asked how she kept appointments, she showed a calendar that she marked every morning. When she got up, she could not tell what day of the week it was, or what year, or what month, or what date. She would ask the person making the appointment to write the numbers on a piece of paper. She then matched these numbers with the calendar numbers and circled the date on the calendar. For the time of the day, she matched the numbers on the appointment card with the numbers on her wristwatch. She was sometimes a little early since she couldn't count the minute lines, but she was never late.

This woman would not let people know that she had this problem until she felt that the person wouldn't make fun of her. For example, she brought a new cookbook to class one day and she was asked, "How do you use it?" "Well," she answered "I don't, but don't tell anyone. I cook what's in the pictures." In order to make sure she gave her daughter the right amount of medication, she would take the daughter back to the doctor after the prescription was filled and ask the doctor to show her how to give the medicine. She said it took the doctor a while to figure out why she was asking him to demonstrate this. But when he figured out her problem, he drew the dosage on a piece of paper and she matched the picture with the pills.

Obviously, this client had—with the help of friends and family—been able to avoid the school situation and learn how to routinize her own life. Consequently, the academic failure had been avoided and she was now quite self-sufficient. It is unlikely that this situation would occur today since children are expected to remain in school and to learn to their potentials. As a result, children often come up against academic failure before it is determined that they have space and time difficulties. A routine, whether imposed by the school or by the family, is needed to provide some boundaries for independent work, play, and learning.

Additional Exposure to Space and Time Vocabulary Markers

These children do not learn the lexical markers denoting spatial and temporal relationships on the basis of routine daily exposures, and consequently they need additional exposure. For example, a parent may put out a child's clothes at night and the next morning tell the child to "get dressed." But the child cannot complete the act because there is too much of a time gap between actions. Many parents of these children have learned that their instructions must be specific and immediately precede the act. Furthermore, parents recognize that instructions often need to be repeated.

Some exasperated parents say it's easier to do the work for the child than try to explain what's wanted or expected. Other parents, who've had similar learning difficulties in school, have found ways to help their children deal with directions and other difficult tasks. One of the most common parental tools is verbal repetition: "Sandy, go buy some milk. Now tell me what you are to do." This technique usually develops as a result of some noncompliance behavior by the child; the parent tries to avoid the problem by asking the child to repeat the directions.

Additional exposure to the space-time lexicon is not as important as the variety of usage and the means of exposure. Since these children are having difficulty attaching the auditory symbol to the event, it's not hard to recognize why reverbalization assists these children. As the child is exposed to the concepts, he or she has a chance to repeat the utterances full of space and time lexicon back to the adult during the event. This helps the child form a relationship between the word and the event. Therefore, the child has successful practice with words and associated events. As the amount of routine and reverbalization increases, the child begins to learn the associations between the bits of information constituting the concept and the representative experience. The reverbalization is eventually faded, and the child verbalizes subvocally and reauditorizes as a learning aid.

Specific Activities for Remediation

A successful activity is one that:

1. linguistically marks an experience in time and space
2. linguistically describes the relationships between and among various space and time markers
3. utilizes material in the child's particular environment
4. provides practice for the child in using the markers.

Determining which concepts to stress is a function of the child's level of space and time development. To determine the level of development, assess the child's use of space and time concepts and select those concepts that the child uses consistently. For example, if the child uses "up," "in," "on," "down," "under," and "before," then the child is using horizontal and early positive vertical dimension terms. So emphasize negative vertical dimension terms (such as "behind") as well as other single dimension terms.

The exact order of facilitation doesn't appear to be as critical as the complexity and manner of presentation. Once the level of complexity is determined, then choose an activity that meets the four criteria. Activities can be chosen from any of these areas: (1) classroom assignments; (2) activities built around interests and hobbies; (3) tasks about classroom routines; (4) travel activities; (5) activities of daily living, such as cooking or dressing; (6) science tasks or experiments; and (7) art tasks, geography lessons, or mapping lessons. The best way to increase exposure and provide a variety of exposure for spatial and temporal terms is to have the child "work through" the activity.

Working through the activity involves:

1. explaining the task using spatial and temporal terms, then having the child describe the task using the same terms;

2. doing each element of the activity according to directions that necessitate space and time markers;
3. reiterating each direction when the direction is completed;
4. repeating the directions or sequence of events for the entire activity. Directions not only require the use of spatio-temporal terms but also require the use of appropriate referents in order for the child's speech act to be referentially clear to the hearer. Therefore, the child's ability to do the activity involves verbally sequencing by correct order of propositional acts, which provides practice and extra exposure in the child's needed verbal mode.

Wilson-Henry and Homchick (1978) developed various forms of activities in which the required skills and levels of difficulty were slightly different. These activities (displayed in Table 6-1) include: sequencing picture cards and telling an appropriate story; anticipating the next logical step of a sequence; relating different stories for one set of picture cards; sequencing the story for one complex picture; sequencing actual items during the making of the item; sequencing school routines; sequencing home and other daily routines; and sequencing spontaneous speaking situations. The difficulty between and among tasks is hierarchical to some extent, with the easiest task listed first and the most difficult task listed last. The difficulty within the tasks is measured by the number of propositions in each activity. Table 6-1 also illustrates the data-taking procedures for determining whether the child's activity had the required number of propositions and whether the response was modeled by the adult.

For each of the activities, the child works through the task by following or imitating models coupled with added semantic cues. The models are gradually faded on the rehearsed tasks, and then the child is exposed to new materials without models. The child should eventually produce the utterances without models or extra attention in the form of semantic cues. The data marks on Table 6-1 indicate whether or not the models and prompts are being faded toward spontaneity. Prompts were considered any attempt to direct the child's attention to the significant perceptual cues.

REMEDIATION PLANNING

After the child's language has been qualitatively analyzed, and standardized tests have been administered, the remediation program may be developed. The goals for this type of therapy should be to improve those skills the child can't do well; that is, to spontaneously converse about a topic and be able to follow the content of another speaker's message.

Table 6-1 Spatio-Temporal Activities and a Data-Taking Methodology

Sequencing Task	Session #	1	2	3	etc.
Sequence picture cards and tell an appropriate story.					
up to 4	number	— —●	●	○	
5 to 8	of		○		
9 plus	propositions				
Anticipate next logical step of a sequence (closure).					
Relate different stories for one set of picture cards.					
Sequence actual items (making an item).					
up to 4					
5 to 8					
9 plus					
Sequence school routine.					
up to 4				—●	
5 to 8					
9 plus					
Sequence home and other daily routines.					
up to 4					
5 to 8					
9 plus					
Sequence spontaneous speaking events.					
up to 4				—	
5 to 8					
9 plus				—●	
Questions and answers.					

Key: — incorrect
   ● correct with a model
   ○ correct without a model

Source: An unpublished case study of a child with spatio-temporal problems. C. Wilson-Henry and A. Homchick, 1978.

Academic Goals

Examples of yearly academic goals for Johnny, the child in the baseball game, might be as follows:

1. Johnny will sequence eight propositions in a spontaneous conversation about a topic he chooses.
2. Johnny will follow the classroom sequence of directions for one week without additional teacher repetitions specifically for Johnny.

Objectives

The objectives should be based on skills that can be improved to meet the child's goals. The ability to converse can be seen as the ability to perform a speech event that would probably consist of several speech acts. Since the spatio-temporal problems are specifically involved with the semantic concepts attached to lexicon, then the speech act is too global a unit of analysis for the problem. The task must be further divided into those parts that reflect the child's ability to perform a speech act. Semantic concepts are part of the proposition (referring and predicating abilities), and the ability to use these concepts effectively depends on the conventional elements shared by speaker and hearer. Therefore, the objectives should emphasize the ability to say something about an object, action, or event (proposition) and then link that idea by space or time to another idea (proposition). The basic problems are the sequencing of the child's ideas and the ability to follow the ordering of another speaker's ideas.

The following objectives have been written for the previously stated goals:

1. Given sequence picture cards, Johnny will tell an appropriate story consisting of four propositions. (The criterion is increased in future objectives, up to approximately nine propositions.)
2. Given an activity (based on a classroom activity, on pictures, or on something he likes to do), Johnny will anticipate the next logical step of a sequence.
3. Given a story for a set of sequence cards, Johnny will tell an appropriate but different story for the same set of cards, beginning with three cards. (Each card should represent at least one idea. As in all of the objectives, the number of ideas is steadily increased.)
4. Given one picture that represents multiple ideas, Johnny will sequence a story beginning with four ideas. (This objective is more difficult than the first three objectives because the ordering of semantic cues from left to right has been eliminated in this task.)
5. Given directions and materials by order of use, Johnny will sequence the making of an item: (a) while doing the making; (b) after the making is completed but the same materials are exhibited so the child has the semantic cues still available; (c) after the immediately available materials are removed; and (d) after all of the semantic visual cues are removed. (This objective is really several daily objectives that utilize techniques

suitable for classroom and/or individual direction. A child who can successfully complete this objective will be using skills necessary for various home and school activities. Again, as the child becomes more proficient the criterion is increased.)

6. Given an activity, Johnny will verbalize the sequence of activities immediately following completion of this activity. (The criterion and the amount of detail required in each step of the sequence depend on the level of the child. And, of course, the level depends on the number of required semantic concepts. Johnny could do one step of a sequence—sometimes two—by chance. For example, "After math (1) we go to recess (2)." The child with spatio-temporal disorders will often separate several activities by a lapse of time between the first activity and the second. For example, "After math we went home." But math is the second classroom subject of the day; therefore, this isn't appropriate sequencing. Calendars and visual prompting by pictures and cards may be necessary to teach this objective. Work on sequencing school activities—Objective 6—and home activities—Objective 7—should begin during the first lesson and increase in difficulty by increasing the propositions. Work on these objectives should begin early because these latter objectives come closest to skills wanted in the final goals.)

7. Given a calendar, Johnny will verbally sequence home routines and, if possible, write the routines into a written story. (The comments under Objective 6 also apply to this objective. This objective may also be broken down for the written tasks.)

8. Johnny will verbally sequence four propositions into a speech event. This objective is really a reduction of Goal 1. Because spontaneous speaking requires internal organization without the aid of visual semantic cues or the routinization of tasks, this objective should be postponed until the child experiences consistent success in all of the other objectives.

9. Given a *who, what, where,* or *when* question in any of the aforementioned objectives, Johnny will respond with the appropriate constituent referent. The criterion is an all-or-none situation. Johnny will be either appropriate or inappropriate. The clinician or educator should begin with the easiest question form and progress to more difficult questions requiring spatial and temporal terminology. Questions that can be answered by a one-word object or event are the easiest. The most difficult questions are those that require answers that must be inferred or deduced from the activity in which the spatio-temporal terms are incorporated. Here is an example from Objective 1: "Which picture comes *first?* This one or this one? Okay. Now which one comes *after* this picture?"

This question-answer objective may be subdivided into other objectives that are aimed at specific terms. Since concept development (not vocabulary) is the ultimate goal, terminology should really be emphasized throughout all of the activities. The same concept should be linguistically tagged by different terminology. For example: "Yes, this picture comes *after* this one. Now tell me, who is coming to school *after* the girl goes into her classroom? Right. Billy is the *last* one to school. He came *after* everyone else? Did anyone come *after* Billy?" Later the same temporal concepts should be emphasized during the making of an item (Objective 5), or in regard to anticipating a logical step (Objective 6), and so forth. The following lists of questions give examples of the types of referents that are possible in this kind of task:

a. *Simple personal and impersonal referents expressed by What*
    1. What refers to the label of an object: What is that?
    2. What refers to action: What are they doing?
    3. What refers to events: What is she doing with the candle?
    4. What refers to present time: What is the date?
    5. What refers to past time: What was yesterday?
    6. What refers to past: What was yesterday?
    7. What refers to future action: What are you going to do?
    8. What refers to future time: What is tomorrow's date?
    9. What refers to ordering of events or directions. These may be marked in the present, past, or future by the verb. Examples include:
       What did you do *first?*
       What did you do *last?*
       What did you do *next?*
       What did you do *before* you came to class?
       What did you do *each time* you went to baseball practice?
    10. What refers to explanation of a sequence of events: What is happening in the story?
    Questions 9 and 10 are the most difficult types.

b. *Personal referents expressed by Who*
    1. Who refers to a specific person: Who is that?
    2. Who refers to a general category of people: Do you know who that person is? or Who is that? (The answer might be mailman.)
    3. Who requires a personal response for action: Who is going to help with the cleaning?
    4. Whose refers to possession: Whose box is this? All of the who forms may be expressed in the present, past, and future tense.

c. *Places of reference expressed by Where*
    1. Where refers to specific places or addresses: Where do you live?
    2. Where refers to the present place of action: Where do you play?
    3. Where refers to past action: Where did you go?

   4. Where refers to future action: Where are you going?
   5. Where refers to the relationship between two objects: Where is the
      map?
   6. Where refers to the position of a person in relationship to an object
      or location: Where is Mary?
   7. Where refers to movement: Where are you moving? (This might be
      in the game of checkers, for example.)
To answer most of the *where* questions requires, at least, rudimentary
sequencing or the understanding of sequencing. Many of the answers require a spatial term such as "next to," "inside," etc.
d. *Time referents usually expressed by When*
   1. When refers to the present: When are you going?
   2. When refers to the past: When did you leave?
   3. When refers to the future: When will you go?
   4. When refers to an event: When did you have time to do that?
   5. When refers to a general action: When are you going to quit smok-
      ing?
e. *Yes/no and is/does questions related to specific semantic concepts*
   1. Time: Did your mom bring you this morning?
          Will you come back next week?
   2. Space: Did you leave your books at home?
          Will you please put your coat in the closet?
   3. Quantity: Did you buy two pens?
          Could you bring your pets next time?
With these types of questions, although answered by a "yes" or "no,"
the answer effectiveness depends on the speaker's and hearer's shared
knowledge base. The more difficult the question, the greater the knowledge base, the broader the semantic concepts included in the question,
and the greater the number of spatial and temporal variables.
f. *Quantity and quality questions using How and Which*
   1. How is used with number: How many children are in your class?
   2. How is used with size: How big is your house?
   3. Which is used with size: Which one is bigger?
   4. Which is used with number: Which one has more?
   5. Which is used with time: Which dog is coming home next?
g. *Questions requiring a conclusion or series of inferences using How and
   Why*
   1. Why did you do that?
   2. How did you do that?
   3. Why are those two girls in the same class?
   4. Why did you take his book?
   5. How did you find the right room?

The difficulty of questions that require conclusions is related directly to the knowledge base, the speaker's ability to linguistically explain or describe, and the number of inferences necessary for deducing a conclusion.

Although the question difficulty may be influenced by the time of the event, the place or position, and/or the semantic relationships, the linguistic complexity is also affected by the *personalness*. Personalness refers not only to whether the referent in question is animate or inanimate; but, if it is animate, personalness refers to the contiguity between the speaker and the answer referent of the question. For a few children, mostly those children who would be diagnosed as emotionally disturbed, questions aimed directly at the hearer threaten the child's personal security. However, for the majority of children with space and time difficulties, the questions about the answerer are the easiest.

The complexity of personalness is related to the child's ability to differentiate herself or himself from the rest of the environment. When this process is undisturbed, the child can easily shift the points of reference. For example, whether the child is "above" or "below" the "top" of the bed, "up" is a direction that is easily discerned. The process normally allows the child to move other objects or people through the same shifting of referents that occurred for the child's self. For example, if the man is going "up" the stairs, which are either "above" or "below" the child, the child is still capable of recognizing that the man is going "up." The ability to follow relationships in the environment or relationships in directions depends on the child's ability to relate these relationships as a shift of referents for the self and for others.

The child with spatio-temporal problems has difficulty making these shifts. The following examples, from a task that involves following directions, illustrates the need to prearrange and organize materials carefully. If the child and adult are seated on the same side of the table, then the referents of position should be the same for each person. The "top" of the paper, the "sides," the "bottom," and so forth are in the same position for the adult and for the child. If the two people are seated across from each other, the reference points for the same piece of paper are different. The "top" of the paper for one person is now the "bottom" of the paper for the other person, the "right" and "left" sides have switched, and so has the "middle" point. Although a common perception of the paper referents relates to the position of the paper to the person, some of these children do not have *common perspective*. For example, suppose an adult is seated across from a child, and a piece of paper is placed directly in front of the child. The child is asked to put his name in the "middle," but he puts the name, Billy, on "top" because that position is the "middle" of the table.

There is the possibility that the child's shifts in points of reference are stylistic preferences unconventional to other native speakers. The following example has been provided by two language clinicians (Wilson-Henry & Homchick, 1978). An eleven-year-old male had appeared to understand or comprehend the term "half" in following directions, because the child could fold a rectangle or square in half either horizontally or vertically. But when the square piece of paper was placed in front of the child at a rotated angle to look like a diamond and the child was asked to fold it in half, he tried to maintain a vertical and horizontal reference point in relationship to himself and the table. So the piece of paper was folded in four triangles with one set of right and left halves which, although feasible, was not the usual paper reference point. The child had not been using the paper as its own referent, but had been using himself as the referent.

A well ordered session may become ineffective, with a few minutes of unstructured, disorganized free talking negating all of the positive steps taken to organize the child's environment. Certain expectations should be clearly identified prior to remediation: (1) Any talking will pertain to the task, so the child is kept on task by expectation and by the educator's technique of verbal redirection; (2) If the child has something to share verbally, then the item should be used as part of the session; that is, the child should write the topic out as a story with each idea enumerated, and then utilize the material at the appropriate level of difficulty for the objectives; and (3) During any task the child is expected to use specific referents to eliminate "fillers" and excessive use of indefinite words.

Table 6-2 lists common spatial, temporal, and quantity terms used in conversations, directions, and storytelling.

SUMMARY

The child with a semantic language disorder that is associated primarily with difficulty in acquiring space and time concepts will evidence language symptoms. These errors will include problems with using specific referents, problems in denoting space and time by appropriate lexicons, and problems in acquiring the quantity skills. Examples of these errors include the following:

- "*You* have to correct *it* and *they* come by and mark it."
  (Illustrates an inability to use specific referents in the agent or recipient positions.)

- "And after recess we go out to recess."
  (Illustrates a basic problem with temporal marking.)

Table 6-2 Common Spatial, Temporal, Quality, and Quantity Terms

Temporal	Quality/Quantity	Spatial
Next	More	Next to
Before	Another	Before
After	Big (-er and -est may be added	After
Into	to this)	On, on top
Soon	Small	In, into
Later	Large	In between
Now	Long	Between
Above	Short	Middle
Yesterday	Medium	Above
Today	Half	Under
Tomorrow	Little	Over
Calendar dates	Specific quantity, ⅓	Below
Months	or more	Corner
Seasons	Few	Bottom
Numerals for years	Many	Inside
Morning	Lots	Outside
Afternoon	Plenty	Side
Evening	Cup, pint, quart, etc.	End
Days	Inch, foot, etc.	In front of
Weeks	Centimeter, meter, kilo-	Behind
Hours	meter, etc.	Beside
Minutes	One-to-one number cor-	Right
Through	respondence	Left
Away from		Through
Toward		High, tall
Sometimes		Upside down
		Together

- "He climbed up on the hill, uh, mountain, or over the mountain."
  (Illustrates a difficulty with spatial relations.)

- "Maybe you'll have a *few* or *many* or *more anyway*."
  (Illustrates problems with quantifiers.)

The symptoms affect the continuity of the child's language, so that tasks requiring storytelling, describing, asking, explaining, and reporting are difficult. The child's comprehension of questions, following directions, and basic listening skills are also affected.

Activities at home, in the classroom, or in language therapy are aimed at increasing the child's ability to perform these tasks. The emphasis of the activities is on learning the concepts, rather than the vocabulary. Verbal redirection, practice, routinization, and reverbalization are important aspects of the remediation program. Although prognosis depends on many factors, the child who is having academic difficulty because of problems related to space and time will progress quickly through this type of remediation program. Data taking in this area of development is based on the competency of the child; that is, whether or not the child can demonstrate the behavior rather than on accuracy or degree of demonstration.

The following language segment was taken from an eleven-year-old child similar to Johnny (the boy who described the baseball game). This segment was obtained after a semester of language therapy. The child was telling a story. Notice that the referents are more specific than in the baseball story and that the temporal aspect of the story is easily followed. Although the child still has some problems to be remediated, the basic ideas are joined in the most difficult task, spontaneous storytelling.

> "So he (the boy), um, hopped in the tub real fast en pushed 'it' out in the water en he started going, going, pretty soon he was out in the middle en he fell asleep. He's just fellin' asleep, floating along. He wasn't scared or anything. He didn't know where he was going, an 'it' en 'it' started waving, waving. En he was sleepin' away ya know, en en he finally . . . en his dad en her mom was lookin' around en they says, oh no what happened to the boy ya know. En they keep lookin' around they couldn't find him. They ask um the next door neighbors ya know en they . . . no one knew about him. So, um, his dad says, I wonder if he went out in the water. En he saw this big old spot, this little spot . . . this little freckle or whatever. En he looked at it. What is that? En he . . . but it was so dark he couldn't see anything. He just . . . way, way, down in the deep. (En) the boy was just thinkin' oh no what happen if I fell in? En the father says, oh I might go see what that spot is so he hopped in his motor boat en took off you see . . . "

Questions

1. Why are space and time difficulties so important to remediation?
2. When a child exhibits difficulties organizing daily activities, why would space and time concepts be tested?
3. What is the relationship between space and time as assessed by a language sample and as assessed by standardized comprehension tests?
4. What other problems are confused with space and time disorders?
5. How does an educator determine which space and time concepts to facilitate?

REFERENCES

Hannah, E. P. *Applied linguistic analysis.* Northridge, Ca.: Joyce Motion Pictures, Co., 1974.

Kahn, J. Relationship of Piaget's sensorimotor period to language acquisition of profoundly retarded children. *American Journal of Mental Deficiency,* 1975, *79,* 640-644.

Lackner, J. R. A developmental study of language behavior in retarded children. *Neuropsychologia,* 1968, *6,* 301-320.

Lenneberg, E. H., Nichols, I. A., & Rosenberger, E. F. Premature stages in language development in mongolism. In D. M. Rioch & E. A. Weinstein (Eds.), *Disorders of Communication.* New York: Hafner Publishing Co., 1969.

Miller, J. F., & Yoder, D. E. An ontogenetic language teaching strategy for retarded children. In R. L. Schiefelbusch & L. L. Lloyd (Eds.), *Language perspectives, acquisition, and retardation.* Baltimore, Md.: University Park Press, 1974.

Morehead, D. M., & Ingram, D. The development of base syntax in normal and linguistically deviant children. *Journal of Speech and Hearing Research,* 1973, *16,* 330-352.

Schauer, M. *Qualitative analysis of retarded vs. normal children's language samples.* Unpublished master's project, Washington State University, 1978.

Wilson-Henry, C., & Homchick, A. *A case study of spatial-temporal problems.* Unpublished manuscript, Washington State University, 1978.

CHAPTER OBJECTIVES

- write a goal for a child with semantic disorders or a general semantic language disorder.

- write appropriate objectives for a child with semantic disorders.

- explain the rationale for any of the techniques suggested.

- list the techniques for remediating each of the semantic disorders described.

- explain data taking procedures for children with semantic problems.

- describe the relationship between syntax, morphology, phonology, and semantics.

- describe three modeling procedures.

- list and describe activities to be used with children who have semantic problems.

- explain application of the techniques to the home setting or other setting.

- list the approach, techniques, and rationale for a child with a semantic language disorder as determined by the qualitative language analysis.

Chapter 7

Remediation Techniques and Activities for Semantic Disorders

The energy of purposive behavior must be synesis,
when a child struggles to find the perfect balance
between meaning to intend and intending to mean.

Each of the semantic disorders described in Chapter 3 will be discussed separately according to specific and general techniques and approaches determined to be effective in remediating that disorder. There is no one approach or program for any group of children, but use of a theoretical basis consistent with the remediation procedures increases the likelihood of effective and efficient language intervention. The activities that follow the techniques and approaches are suggested as *springboards* to help clinicians and/or educators generate novel ideas tailored to their own situation.

AUDITORY MISPERCEPTION

A child who occasionally evidences auditory misperception errors would probably not be considered for language therapy since this disorder would not affect message effectiveness or academic performance. Occasional errors in auditory perception would be corrected verbally, as they occur, and this would be considered part of the child's overall language program.

In cases where the child's auditory perception and/or integration is assumed to be distorted, then visual cueing would serve as a learning aid for the child. Visual cueing might be provided by orthographic representations (writing out the words) or by a symbol-sign system such as presented with the Rebus Materials (1973). By the same token, these children are often helped once they acquire basic auditory-to-visual reading skills. These cueing efforts are incorporated into the child's classroom, home, or therapy activities by teachers, parents, and/or clinicians.

It is important to complete the association of the visual symbol with the auditory symbols. Therefore, whatever visual cues are provided, the child should be encouraged to produce the corrected production. Until the child says the correction, the input is not likely to have any lasting effect. For example, suppose the child repeatedly uses "brections" for "directions." The letters "br" are written on a card placed next to the syllable "dir." The child's face is directed to the speaker's mouth on the first production and to the written symbol on the second production; then the child is asked to say the syllables as part of the corrected words.

OFF TARGET RESPONDING

Unlike auditory misperceptions, off target responding is a problem that can be remediated directly and effectively. The child's prerequisite skills for responding include (1) identification of a common referent; (2) selective attending to the preceding message and environmental cues; (3) basic comprehension of semantic relations for understanding the established joint references; and (4) basic comprehension of the speaker-to-hearer roles, whether for constituent or yes/no questions or conversational dialogue. Based on the prerequisite level, the clinician or teacher will select the appropriate place for intervention. Each of the above four points will be considered in order to determine the prerequisite level.

Determining Prerequisite Level

At what level is the child able to identify a common referent? The possibilities would include the following: people, objects, actions, events, conditional or causal relations (if . . . then); inferred items; places or locations, space and time for events. By asking a series of questions proceeding from those easiest to answer (what plus object) to the more difficult items (if . . . then why . . .), the clinician is able to determine at what level the child no longer responds appropriately. A list of some of the possible question types was provided in Chapter 6.

Does the child exhibit nonverbal behavior indicative of selective attending? The nonverbal behavior would include appropriate eye contact or observation and no distracting behavior such as playing with fingers, twirling pencils, rocking, and so forth. The child may need to be redirected (verbally or nonverbally) to the referent in order to hear the conversation or attend to the environmental referents for more appropriate responding.

Does the child have enough knowledge about necessary semantic relations to make appropriate utterances about the environment? Semantic relations may be assessed by manipulating environmental objects in conjunction with the child's use of spontaneous language (McLean & Snyder-McLean, 1978). If the child does not have the basic semantic relations, the clinician should go back to establish this knowledge before trying to decrease the frequency of certain language aberrations.

Is the child capable of switching roles between speaker and hearer? Children must be able to demonstrate that they are capable of switching roles, so they can initiate as well as respond appropriately. If a child can't switch roles a pragmatic disorder is present, and it deserves priority attention over the semantic problems.

Once the level of prerequisites has been determined, the remediation approach might include question-and-answer tasks, sequence story tasks, sequence activities as described in Chapter 6, and free conversation activities. The level of prerequisites determines the level of semantic input and/or whether prerequisites should also be established before working on the off target responding.

Question-and-Answer Tasks

The purpose of a question-and-answer task is to determine whether the child is attending to the semantic cues of the environment, to which semantic cues the child is attending, and whether or not the child can put the knowledge into linguistic form.

If a question is answered appropriately and completely, it is assumed that the child's semantic knowledge sufficiently overlaps that of the person asking the question, and that the child can sort this knowledge and represent the answer in linguistic form. For example: "What did you have for lunch?" "Milk and a sandwich." The answer, "Milk and a sandwich" is appropriate and complete unless the hearer knows otherwise. If the child's answer is close to the topic or on the topic of lunch but not completely appropriate, then the child has some overlapping knowledge and is capable of doing some sorting of semantic cues. Suppose that to the question, "Johnny, did you come on the bus this morning?" the child answers, "My mama has a new car." This utterance does not answer the question sufficiently, so now the clinician must use the cues and the technique of verbal redirection to help the child arrive at the appropriate answer to the specific question.

The following segment illustrates the process of verbal redirection that may be used in any setting to assist remediation of an off target utterance:

1. "Joshua, did you come on the bus this morning?"

2. "My mommy has a new car." (The adult recognizes the common elements between the question and the child's answer. In this case, the common element appears to be a mode of transportation.)
3. "Oh, you came in your mother's new car?" (If the adult does not recognize the intent of the child's utterance, which was probably to tell about the new car, then the child will again miss the referent of the question and the response will be off target.)
4. "Yes." (The adult has an appropriate answer and now redirects the child.)
5. "So, you didn't come by bus; you came by car." (The adult asks the original question.) "Did you come on the bus this morning?"

By repeating the entire question after having the answer presented in a dialogue form, the child gains knowledge of the semantic rules underlying this speech act (series of speech acts). The child also receives practice in performing successful speech acts and practice in attending closely to the original referent. If the child begins to sort, attend, and perform speech acts, then the child will not be responding off topic.

Sequence Story Tasks

The sequence story task is another activity with the same goal of learning the semantic rules that underlie the specific speech acts. The objectives center around skills of the speech act performance: sequencing propositions, using and comprehending semantic information, and verbally and nonverbally directing the listening and speaking.

Sequencing becomes more difficult as the number of propositions increases. So the clinician begins with a single proposition and adds another proposition until the speech event is accomplished. The criterion is whether or not the child produces the propositions. Progress is noted by the number of appropriate propositions in a sequence.

A sequence story task that uses pictures to tell a story provides material for a variety of novel utterances for each picture in the sequence. If the child's utterance has the appropriate content and is performed with the essential elements, then the child is performing a speech act. The adult uses appropriate verbal and nonverbal cues to direct the child to the next picture of the sequence. If the child errs in the sequencing of the propositions (even though each utterance may be singularly appropriate for each of the pictures), the child should be redirected back through the sequence. An example of appropriate utterances (that is, the utterances match the pictures) but inappropriate propositions would be: "The boy is going to the store. He has a wagon." An example of redirection follows. Notice that the adult tries to connect or associate the two utterances rather than ignore the inaccurate utterances or model an utterance to be imitated.

> "Is the boy using the wagon to go to the store?"
> "No."
> "What is he doing with the wagon?"
> "He's carrying the groceries."
> "He's carrying groceries in his wagon?" (Again the adult tries to associate the ideas.)
> "Yes."
> "Then let's tell the story. The boy went to the store, and then he carried his groceries home in his wagon. Now you tell it."

As emphasized in the question-and-answer tasks, the verbal redirection and reworking of an idea provides the child with successful performances of speech acts as speech events. The performance also provides a chance to sort and learn the available semantic information.

Additional materials for the sequence story task include (1) academic activities, such as direction learning; (2) routine activities (such as "What did you do today?") that are carried out by verbal directions and redirections; (3) calendar activities, such as "When do you get summer vacation?"; (4) home activities, such as the sequencing involved in cooking, building, cleaning, etc.; (5) play activities (particularly with rules) such as baseball, checkers, etc.; (6) arts and crafts, such as "How do you make a pumpkin for Halloween?"

The following activity is presented to illustrate that any activity can be used to facilitate appropriate semantic and pragmatic language acquisition.

> *Adult:* "You've done a good job today. Next time (points to calendar) we are going to do something special. We are going to carve pumpkins. What shall I bring?"
> *John:* "Pumpkins!"
> *Adult:* "How many?"
> *Amy:* "Five!"
> *Adult:* "Why do we need five pumpkins?"
> *Sarah:* "One for Mike, Amy, me, and you."
> *Adult:* "Do John and Allen each get one?"
> *Sarah:* "Yes!"
> *Adult:* "How many pumpkins is that?"
> *Amy:* "Don't know!"
> *Adult:* "Let's count it together." (counts) "How many do we need?"
> *Unison:* "Six."
> *Adult:* "What else will we need?"

Sarah: "A face."

Adult: "A face? Why do we need a face? Here is my face and you have a face." (touches Sarah's face)

Mike: (Gets nervous) "Well, I mean I'm going to be a ghost." (off topic)

Adult: "We'll talk about what we will wear for Halloween but" (redirection) "the question was 'What shall I bring next time to carve pumpkins?' "

Sarah: "Six pumpkins!"

Adult: (She has the visual cues to use and puts a paper pumpkin out in front of each child.) "Okay, I'll bring six pumpkins."

Mike: "Not like this—"

Adult: "What's wrong, Mike?"

Mike: "This isn't a pumpkin to cut."

Adult: "Do you want a different kind of pumpkin for carving?"

Allen: "Yeah—like this." (holds his hands up in a round form)

Adult: "Allen, shall I hold the paper up?" (She holds the paper up.)

Mike: "No, I want a pumpkin from the store."

Adult: "What kind of store?" (pulling in details to link ideas)

Sarah: "A Safeway store."

Adult: "What kinds of things do we buy at a Safeway kind of store?" (More details are added and thus the semantic cues are being associated.)

Allen: "Hamburger, hot dogs, soap."

Sarah: "Dog food!"

Mike: "Potato chips and ice cream."

Amy: "I like the 'spadette'!"

Adult: "You like spaghetti? Well, we could buy the spaghetti at the stores that are like Safeway." (redirection) "What else would we buy at the store, Amy?"

Mike: "Uh, uh, uh (important!!!) This guy's Dad works there!"

Adult: "Amy was going to tell me about the things to buy at a store like Safeway, and you believe that his (points) Dad works there?"

Mike: "He lives next door." (The child is going on without staying on the topic.)

Adult: "Who is this person, Mike? Tell me *his* (points) name."

Mike: "Allen."

Adult: "So, Allen's dad works at Safeway. He works at a grocery store, Mike. What would you buy from Allen's dad at the store?"

Mike: "All sorts of stuff."

Adult: "Yes, we could buy all kinds of food, groceries, vegetables . . . . Could we buy pumpkins at the grocery store?"

Sarah: "Yes!"
Adult: "Sarah, what shall I bring next time and where shall I get them?"

It would be good to go through the event with different phrasing to establish the sequencing of where the pumpkins would be purchased and when the activity of carving the pumpkins would take place. It would also be more effective to go through the actual sequencing involved in the pumpkin carving. This particular activity took place in a preschool. Any active process can serve as a sequence activity for language facilitation. To promote continuity between sessions, it is important to repeat what occurred at the previous session and in the immediate class period. All activities should have the goal of helping the child use the meaningful environmental information to affect a hearer.

Therefore, the off topic problem may be remediated through activities that help the child follow the referential meaning by using simple techniques such as redirection, reverbalization, and practice of appropriate on-topic situations. Although extra practice may be provided by activities and materials that are easily selected from daily situations and applied to therapeutic settings; teachers and parents also find these techniques easy to use. Once the environment is consistent, then the remediation process is greatly enhanced.

SYNTACTIC ERRORS

A syntactic error, as defined in Chapter 3, represents an underlying confusion in the child's semantic basis. Activities and techniques designed to remediate or improve the underlying semantic skills are appropriate for the word order problems. Problems related to the morphological acquisition of inflectional endings, such as *-ed* for past regular tense, usually do not affect word order. However, many children who exhibit the problems discussed in this chapter also develop the morphophonemic rules. These rules govern which types of sounds may be added to alter the meaning. For example, when a word ends in a voiced consonant, the plural is made by adding a voiced consonant, *-s,* so "dog" becomes "dogs" in which the *-s* is pronounced as a *-z.* Because this type of morphological development affects the surface structure, a description of modeling is provided so that the adult is always facilitating the child's linguistic forms even though the primary objectives are designed to meet other therapeutic needs.

As the child develops a thorough knowledge of the perceptual and functional attributes that constitute the content, the structural skills or linguistic forms representing this knowledge may be taught through modeling procedures. With modeling, the adult produces an utterance with a rising intonation pattern and with a structural complexity slightly above the child's linguistic level (as determined by the results of the quantitative language tests). The child is expected to imitate this utterance as closely as possible. Once the model has been made and/or the child makes a production, the adult then has several options that will assist in encouraging the dialogue. The options include (1) expanding the child's utterances; (2) producing another utterance that brings new information into the present topic; (3) responding to the child's utterance as if the utterance were a speech act intended to alter the hearer's attitudes, beliefs, or behaviors; and/or (4) going through a question-and-answer task to encourage the child to produce a similar utterance in the same situation. At any point in the dialogue, the modeling options described here and in the literature are available for application (e.g., Cazden, 1972; Lee, 1975; Muma, 1970).

The following examples depict each of these four options during an attempt to model for the child. Option 1, an expansion of the child's utterance, is an adult's utterance which is more structurally complex, but does not add new information to the basic message: "Washington, where's your daddy?" "Daddy go work." "Oh, your daddy went to work." The notion of expansion is quite similar to the natural parent technique described in the literature (Brown & Bellugi, 1964; Cazden, 1972; Muma, 1970). With Option 2, the expansion of the child's utterance may be more complex semantically, thus adding new information. The child might say, "That my doll." The adult could add information by saying, "Yes, your doll is sitting on my desk." It should be noted that most utterances that add new semantic content are also expansions. This is not unexpected since it has already been suggested that increases in expressed ideas also increase the surface structure.

Option 3 is one of the most effective options available to the adult. The adult responds to whatever is the assumed intent of the child's utterance, pairing this response with the verbal explanation. The adult's verbal modeling may be an expansion with or without new semantic ideas, but the verbalizations are occurring in context and there's a purpose for continuing the verbal exchange (Chapter 8).

Option 4 is a usage variation of the models suggested previously. This option is actually a technique used to incorporate the various models into an exchange between a speaker and a hearer. The child is asked a question and is given an opportunity to verbalize either through nonverbal or verbal means. For example, "Please tell me about your picture." The child responds; the adult responds again with another opportunity, followed by expansion, followed by reaction, and so forth.

This last option really becomes a series of questions (verbal and nonverbal) followed by answers (models) to which either the adult or child responds. The adult eventually reinstates the initial question. For example: "Cindy, where's your shoe?" "My shoe not there." "Your shoe isn't here, but where is it?"

"Don't know." "You don't know? Maybe it is in your closet." The child finds her shoe and the adult resets the initial question: "Where was your shoe?" The child says, "In closet." The adult again has the option: "Your shoe was in the closet. Tell me where you found your shoe." At this point it is possible to begin a direct imitation or complete imitation. Through this question-and-answer exchange, the child is given the necessary practice in following the topic and in using more complex structures.

Modeling is maximally effective during the transitory period of linguistic development, when the child's language changes from productions representative of semantic relations to more grammatical forms similar to adult structures. If a school-age child has difficulty with only the linguistic formulation, then the child is probably a second language learner or has dialectical interference that would probably benefit from drill on the representative or desired forms. Even if the child has a basic knowledge of semantic concepts, the child must also have knowledge of time, space, quantity, and quality, or the modulations will be affected. For example, plurals are marked when the child makes the distinction between "one" and "more" and not because the child has learned the adult's perspective of a rule. If the child can't mark the distinction, but has the semantic knowledge (as may be the case with second language and dialectical learners), then drills on -s, -z, -iz may be profitable. However, the models and drills alone will not eliminate a syntactic (word order) problem that stems from a lack of semantic development or from a semantic disorder.

Recent research results (Lucas, 1977; Mundell & Lucas, 1978) regarding intervention suggest that if a child's semantic acquisition is improved for adequate pragmatic development, then the structural development will also continue to improve. However, the converse relationship is not as easily predicted; that is, structural drills do not necessarily improve a child's ability to use language to change attitudes, beliefs, or behaviors of a hearer. Therefore, syntactic errors as described in Chapter 3 have a semantic basis that may be dealt with by facilitating the child's semantic and pragmatic skills. The semantic-pragmatic intervention often results in an increase in grammatical and syntactical acquisition.

Therefore, the same activities and techniques described in Chapter 6 should alleviate word order problems since these activities foster referential clarity as expressed through conventional ordering of the semantic relations. If this approach is not helpful, then the child (expected chronological age two to five) needs direct experience with the environment to facilitate basic semantic relations representing the linearity of the English language. During these experiences, models (marking) provide practice with the linguistic code. Data are based on which semantic relations and functions are being facilitated. Again, the child either demonstrates knowledge or does not; there's no way to assume partial accuracy by a percentage. Therefore a basic goal might be written as follows: *The child will demonstrate the semantic relations and semantic functions when given a structured environment designed to necessitate use of the relations and functions.*

Objectives would be written for each of the semantic relations to be fostered. It is crucial that the adult realizes that ideas, not constructions, are being facilitated. Therefore, the pragmatic suggestions for techniques in Chapter 8 should be followed.

By working directly on the underlying semantic relations, and/or on the concomitant language disorders related to syntactic errors, and/or on the surface representation, the child should show progress. The pace of progress will vary, depending a great deal on whether the problem is a semantic delay, disorder, or structural style preference. It is often most difficult to obtain consistent improvement with the style preference condition because it is not related to the semantic skills but to the child's environment.

SEMANTIC WORD ERRORS

The semantic word errors are usually related to time, space, quantity, and/or quality terms. Since these words organize the child's environment, the purpose of therapy is to provide visual cues in small increments of increasing difficulty to improve these basic concepts. Although Chapter 6 dealt in depth with this problem, some comments regarding general vocabulary development will be considered at this time.

Chapter 1 described the current theoretical position concerning semantic lexical development. Results from therapeutic experience support the idea that vocabulary acquisition is a gradual process reflective of the child's cognitive development. For example, the child who misses a vocabulary item on a comprehension test may be overheard using the word in context outside the testing situation; or the child who is drilled on picture cards may be able to give the correct label for each picture but never use the vocabulary item in conversation. It is also quite apparent that children will define, and use, vocabulary items as their exposure or background permits. Thus the eight-year-old child who tells the teacher that his father has been "requested" rather than "sequestered" for jury duty is trying to use words that he has heard in context but for which he doesn't have an adult dictionary-like meaning.

Providing activities and tasks for vocabulary development or enrichment should be based on the child's corresponding level of cognitive development. Children between the ages of zero and two (chronological language and mental ages are assumed to be the same) learn from being manipulated and from manipulating their environment through sensory and motor input and function. So for vocabulary acquisition, these children should be exposed to sensory experiences that can be manipulated motorically to facilitate the development of necessary information. During this time, the caretaker should be marking the experiences with lexical tags, using rising inflectional patterns for encouraging verbal responses from the child, and talking in short but grammatical utterances. These parental guides are the same techniques that the educator or clinician should be using constantly with these children.

As the child's experiences grow, he or she begins to verbalize about those experiences. The first verbalizations are related to a self-interest perspective, followed by those that are part of a concerted effort to share information. This process of incorporating others into the child's own interests usually occurs between the ages of two and seven. So a child whose vocabulary growth and/or mental age corresponds to this period needs experiences that are meaningful, so that the child may acquire enough content or knowledge to use the vocabulary concepts as self-intended. Even adults often require additional experiences with the same abstract notion in order to understand the concept enough to use it even in the most limited manner.

Like the adult, the child needs experiences that are flexible and not limited. For example, a giraffe and an elephant are limited concepts and usually have mostly nonfunctional meanings for handicapped children. However, experiences in which everyday objects are used in a variety of ways provide the extra exposure and learning time required by the child with special needs. The notion of using environmental objects often seems difficult and abstract to an adult—and it should! Children and adults do not think alike, and an adult task does little for a child's needs. Here are some suggestions for learning to use a daily object or event:

1. Pick any object already in the child's environment, such as a brush.
2. What are the perceptual features or attributes of that object? Brushes have bristles that are soft, hard, stiff; they are different shapes and sizes; some have long handles, etc.
3. What are the functional attributes? Brushes brush hair—my hair, your hair, dog's hair; or the bristles can be pushed; or the brush can be washed, shaken, cleaned, etc. The brush is an instrument, recipient of action, object of action, etc.
4. If the child is beyond the basic semantic relations expressed by two and three terms, add more variety by increasing the number and type of brushes available for inspection. Put the brushes into context by placing them in housekeeping, hygiene, or health science areas.
5. Since the child should be approaching a sharing (rather than an egocentric) conversational level, provide multiple opportunities for a variety of speech acts. (See Chapter 8 regarding the opportunities.)

By using the above principles, the child's language is allowed to function while the language base is increased. The child uses the language to meet needs, and the adult incorporates a variety of concepts that are being presented in meaningful associations with child-oriented experiences. Again, modeling techniques provide an opportunity for the child and the adult to exchange the linguistic lead in a given context. The more opportunities to participate in experiences using the concepts, the more likely the concepts will be learned. The child who is seven and has the syntax, morphology, and phonology of a seven year old, has enough oral language skills to be an effective communicator even though advanced semantic concepts continue to expand through adulthood.

The elementary school-age child is engaged in learning the space, time, quality, and quantity words that run parallel to academic progress and achievement. The school-age child's vocabulary definitions are related more to the child's organization of daily experiences. A four-year-old would have defined "bike" as "Billy's got a yellow bike and he rides it." The same child at eight or nine years of age would relate the bike to specific experiences, but group some standard characteristics of all bikes (such as "you ride 'em to school and they've got pedals, two wheels," etc.). A child at this age is ready for categorization, a task more akin to an adult method of thinking than to a youngster's thinking pattern.

Several language intervention programs ask the child to do categorization tasks (such as "Put the foods together" or "Which pieces are furniture?") before the child has the prerequisites. Categorization tasks should begin only after the child has language skills comparable to the seven year old, and thus is beginning to define (an adult task) by grouping characteristics.

By the time the child has learned to categorize—which also indicates that the child has learned other systematic ways to deal verbally with the environment—the child is ready for adultlike reasoning. Defining words, drawing conclusions, making inferences, abstracting from line drawings, learning by being told abstract rules, and other adult methods may be utilized. The child who can do these tasks has a mental age of approximately eleven.

Before discussing the next semantic disorder and the treatment possibilities, a few comments regarding materials for children are warranted. Although handicapped children often need more exposure and more experiences than children who are acquiring language skills in their normal environment, this difference does not mean that the handicapped child will think or process more like an adult. Even the most distractible four year old needs a variety of semantic cues for acquiring knowledge and for learning to represent the knowledge in linguistic code.

Once the environment is reduced to sterile one-to-one line representations, line drawings, or even activity line drawings, the task becomes more concrete to the adult and more abstract to the child. Arranging the environment for maximum attending does not mean sterilizing the setting. Controlling the environment means maximizing the child's learning set by organizing the stimuli; by providing materials at the child's cognitive level for maximum interest; by providing opportunities for performing speech events (see Chapter 8); by allowing for maximum total growth of the child in all areas—including social, emotional, cognitive, motor, and linguistic abilities; by allowing the social/environmental aspects to reinforce the child rather than using artificial, abstract, linguistic verbals such as "Good, boy!"; and by being accountable for real changes in the child's behavior, not just for numbers on charts.

If the child's attending behavior is a concern, then the adult should provide materials and activities at the child's level of attending and provide an incompatible behavior to take the place of the child's inattentive behavior. Often, when language is increased, some of the negative behaviors do temporarily increase, but then these taper off as the language takes the place of the attention-getting or self-stimulatory behavior.

The following example illustrates the importance of presenting materials and activities that are semantically appropriate for the child. Six handicapped four-year-old children are grouped together because each child is at least two-and-a-half years delayed. This piece of information suggests that the most complex language that each child uses is equal to that of an 18-month-old child or perhaps less. But because the children look like four-year-old children and because the teacher thinks like an adult, the children are asked to identify pictures of animals. The adult is also tuned into defining as a task that is concrete to an adult; so each child is told, "Say what the animal says." In this way, the child labels "cow" and defines the "cow" by the word "moo."

In the previous example, have the children been given extra experiences that would enable them to use the word "cow" or any other animal vocabulary in a functional manner? Of course not. Has the teacher capitalized on the perceptual and functional attributes the child should be learning? No. If a child can distinguish a cow from a horse, there's some sorting and discriminating being done. An activity that increases, stimulates, and challenges this sorting will increase the child's knowledge. If animals are meaningful to a child at this mental age, it is because of the child's experiences with hearing, seeing, and smelling the animals. So, if this topic is relevant, put the animals into a context and TALK! Those perceptual and functional attributes must be linguistically marked for the child. Once the experience is established and the opportunities for learning are provided, the adult must learn to LISTEN! The child doesn't want to label and define; the child prefers to tell, even in jargon, about the animal being held, the things the animal does, what the animal eats, etc. Use the child's environment to maximize the learning. Put aside the adult's environment which tends to be too abstract for most language disordered and language delayed children.

The preceding points about activities regarding semantic development of lexicon might be summarized and listed as follows:

1. If the child is using language below the two-year-old level, activities and materials to maximize vocabulary enrichment should provide sensory input and motor expression. The techniques should be based on modeling with rising patterns for response. Methods for withholding materials, facilitating participation, and recording responding will be discussed in Chapter 8.

2. The child who is two to seven in language development needs materials related to personal experiences. Activities that involve making, doing, and playing with real objects allow for exposure and practice. Only after considerable language development (approximately that of a four to five year old) is the child ready for pictures as teaching devices. Pictures that represent the real experiences do teach tasks and labels; but without the experiences, the abstraction is adultlike and the child can't relate to the picture for spontaneous usage.

   Since vocabulary development is usually part of an overall program to improve many of the child's language abilities, goals would be directed toward the child's use of the language, and the objectives would emphasize vocabulary development. An objective for specific lexicon should represent the semantic concepts. For example, "LeAnne will use the listed terms appropriately during a ten-minute activity of questions and answers." The terms might be "seed," "stem," "leaf," "flower," "dirt," "soil," "ground," "water," "sunlight," "food." The questions and answers refer to a follow-up exchange after LeAnne has had experience with these ideas or concepts. If the child only needs vocabulary development, the child is a second-language learner and/or is from a different sociocultural environment. Otherwise, there would be other priority problems, such as space and time problems.

3. Children who have the language skills of a seven year old or greater are learning to expand on previously acquired vocabulary and are making greater use of space and time concepts for organization. Therefore therapy will follow the suggestions presented in Chapter 6 or those techniques adults use to acquire new vocabulary. Semantic word errors may exist, and thus therapy may take a number of different approaches all aimed at improving the child's use of semantic concepts or lexicon. The techniques and data taking depend on the skills being facilitated. Prognosis is a function of the extent of disorder and/or deficits in concept building, as well as a function of the child's ability to learn and use these ideas.

WORD-FINDING PROBLEMS

If a child's difficulties in using words are really a result of recall problems, then activities or tasks to facilitate recall may be utilized. These types of activities are outlined in the literature on aphasia (as cited in Chapter 3). Examples of recall facilitation tasks include (1) fill-in or completion activities in which the child is given a leading utterance (such as "We eat ———") and the child is to finish or complete the utterance; (2) association activities between ideas ("What goes with bacon?" or "Bacon and ———"); (3) descriptive tasks in which the child is taught to think of associations or alternate words that would describe the item; and (4) activities that categorize by units to provide a semantic mental set (as exemplified by topic utterances, "Today we'll talk about the *supermarket*").

Some children who appear to have word-finding difficulties are not experiencing problems with recall but with meaning or concepts. For example, children with space and time difficulties will use fillers such as "um" or "uh" as well as indefinite terms such as "it" or "anytime," which *color* the language with the appearance of word-finding difficulties. It's the author's experience that the majority of older language disordered children experience more difficulty with meaning than with actual recall processing. Furthermore, techniques to facilitate the development of meaning of general vocabulary and of specific space, time, and quantity terms decrease the linguistic problems associated with word finding. By acquiring more knowledge about the concepts represented by the lexicon, the child has fewer choices and therefore has less difficulty selecting the words.

Therefore, with the exception of some word-finding techniques suggested for recall facilitation, the word-finding techniques suggested in this chapter are based on the rationale that the symptoms characterize semantic disorders already discussed. Therefore, the techniques and data taking suggested for spatio-temporal problems are facilitating vocabulary development and will alleviate word-finding symptoms, unless the disorder is with recall.

NEOLOGISMS

The construction of neologisms is again a symptom of a more general semantic language disorder that should be the primary focus of therapy. However, certain neologisms may be repeated consistently, which indicates that techniques to disrupt the pattern may be desirable. For the phonological neologism, use the same visual cueing techniques suggested for auditory misperceptions. It is important to ask the child to verbalize the visual input so that the association between the auditory (oral to aural) and the intervention modality (visual) is provided. The auditory pattern produced by the child may not be disrupted by auditory or visual correction without the child producing the new pattern vocally or subvocally. Asking the child to repeat the utterance is a good technique for many language disorders—particularly when teachers, clinicians, and parents have first tried the auditory correction, have asked the child to read the correction, and then have gone back to repeating the corrected pattern. The correct production is facilitated by visual cues. Although reducing neologisms and auditory misperceptions may be immediate objectives, with reduced frequency being the criterion, these errors would be secondary to a communication goal.

PHONOLOGICAL DISORDERS

The child who is omitting functors and syllables in speech needs the rules for combining sound symbols with morphemes. The connection between phonology and morphology is based on a rule-governed system that is included as part of the essential rule components of speech acts. This child's unintelligibility is greatly reduced when patterns representative of the rules are emphasized in remediation. As previously mentioned, there are several approaches for remediation that deal directly with phonology. The inclusion of this problem under semantic disorders illustrates another perspective: Provide patterns or examples of the morphophonemic rules to remediate the omission of syllables and functors, since this omission represents a breakdown in semantic expression.

The patterning approach was originally the result of observations made during diagnostic evaluations. Children who experience a problem with combining morphemes do better on direct imitation tasks than on tasks involving elicited imitation or production. This observation led therapists to provide sentences at or below the child's linguistic level for direct imitation. The patterning approach was much more effective than work on specific sound syllables, articulation, or grammatical aspects. With direct imitation, the child is first expected to include all syllables. Then the child's overall intelligibility is emphasized by models and repetitions in the context of a child and adult interchange. The same phrases from the sentences are then used in restricted stories or conversations.

Only children who are able to express all semantic relations and functions as well as all types of speech acts should be given pattern experiences. Furthermore, these children should not evidence any other semantic disorders except for the problem with intelligibility.

TOPIC OR REFERENT IDENTIFICATION

A child cannot be a consistently effective communicator if he or she cannot identify the topic or referent in the hearer's or speaker's utterances. The steps to follow to develop skills in referent or topic identification are listed below:

1. Provide an experience or setting that ensures joint reference between the speaker and hearer, since the child's or adult's outside experiences may

not be fully understood or expressed. For example, suppose the child says, "I picked flowers yesterday." The adult has to acknowledge this information as accurate since the adult wasn't with the child and doesn't know if the child did indeed pick flowers. If the adult says, "We're going to talk about going shopping," it is assumed that the shopping experiences of the adult are similar to the shopping experiences of the child.

2. Provide key ideas, vocabulary, or points regarding the experience or setting. Key points, ideas, and/or vocabulary may be provided by pictures, picture story charts, question constituent charts, and/or story charts with sentences (for older children). Examples of the visual aids are shown in Figure 7-1. Visual aids like these are found in most classrooms for the preschool, kindergarten, or first-grade child. For the younger children, use the pictures and objects on the chart rather than the written sentence or words. These charts may be written as the children are directed through the ideas and/or they may be created before the children arrive.

Figure 7-1 Examples of Vocabulary Story Charts

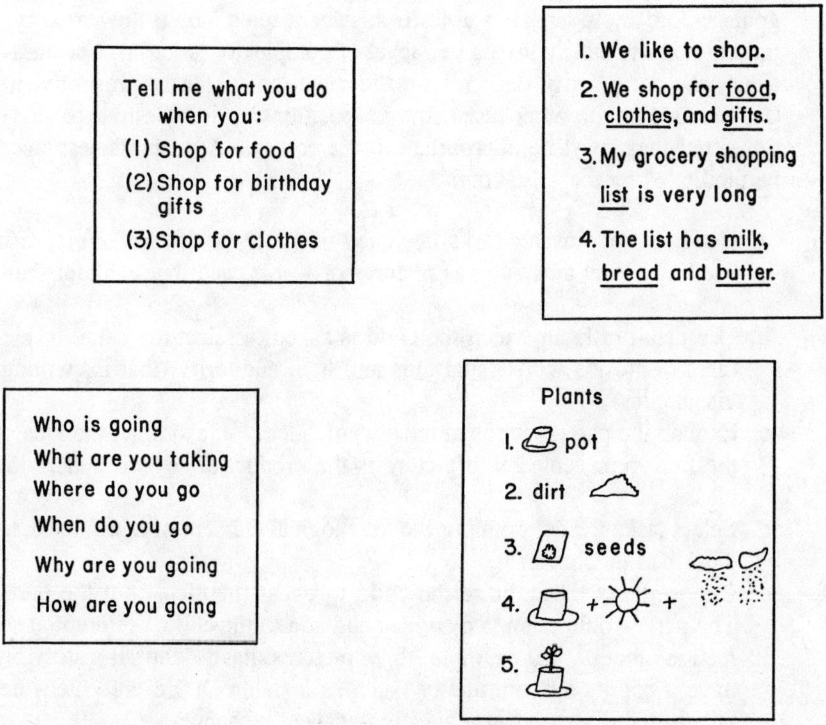

Tell me what you do
when you:
(1) Shop for food
(2) Shop for birthday gifts
(3) Shop for clothes

1. We like to shop.
2. We shop for food, clothes, and gifts.
3. My grocery shopping list is very long
4. The list has milk, bread and butter.

Who is going
What are you taking
Where do you go
When do you go
Why are you going
How are you going

Plants
1. pot
2. dirt
3. seeds
4. + +
5.

3. Present the key ideas, points, and/or vocabulary before the activity. Then teach by means of the activity, and reinforce with questions and repetitions after the activity.

4. Activities should be at the child's cognitive and/or academic and educational level and representative of interests and daily concerns. For example, an activity for an eight-year-old boy who builds model airplanes at home might involve talking about the making of a paper airplane and how it is similar or different to building model aircraft.

5. Since referent identification involves a sorting of attributes and linguistic decoding, followed by expression of the identification, it is critical to model appropriate utterances regarding the activity so the child can hear and compare self-produced utterances against the adult's utterances. In other words, the adult should talk through the activity before the activity begins and again after the activity is finished.

6. The child is expected to reiterate the clinician's utterances as well as produce novel utterances about the activity. A question-answer-question format facilitates listening and keeps the child on topic during the activity. As with the other semantic disorders, the goal is appropriate language usage based on acquisition of semantic rules. Intermediate or academic goals would include being able to answer a question, follow a story, present a story, etc., with a given level of complexity (criteria). For questions, the complexity depends on the question variables presented in Chapter 6. For the other tasks, the propositions are the desired productions, but they must be appropriate to the context. Appropriateness may be facilitated by the following:

   a. Use question-answer tasks designed to elicit specific referents, first cued by visual aids such as pictures or words, and then without these aids.

   b. Use detail tasks in which the child is asked to select the detail in pictures or stories with visual aids and then auditorily (that is, without visual cues).

   c. Explain the parts that constitute a whole idea. For example, the idea of the farm represented in a picture is the product of several underlying ideas.

   d. Select tasks for determining the next logical element of a sequence, as described in Chapter 6.

   e. Choose tasks that require the child to guess the idea from the parts. The parts would complete an idea and add to the child's referential selection process. For example, three pictures that do not tell a story but have a common denominator (such as a "store") are presented, detailed, and discussed in a question-answer exchange.

Objectives would emphasize the types of tasks outlined above, with the desired goal being the appropriate usage of referents and/or the appropriate identification of a speaker's referents. The criteria are based on the percentage of appropriate versus inappropriate referents, as judged by the adult speaker, during a given time or a given assessment activity (apart from times of correction or therapy).

TOPIC CLOSURE

A child who verbalizes incessantly can be as frustrating as the nonverbal child. In order to decrease the talking, several changes should be made: (1) the child should be made aware of the linguistic markers indicating the topic; (2) the child should be cued to recognize the boundaries of the topic; and (3) the child should be cued to recognize the content of what he or she has spoken.

Closure techniques involve cueing the child verbally and visually as to when and what to say in an open-ended situation. Open-ended situations allow the opportunity to include new information. Examples of verbal openers include: "Tell me about your weekend." or "What do you think about the picture?" or "What do you think the story is about?" or "What do you like to do during vacation?" The answers to these questions really have no beginning or end. However, most speakers know intuitively when enough has been said about the topic. The child with the topic closure problem doesn't have the essential boundary elements of speech acts and cannot determine when an utterance has had maximum impact on the hearer. With these children, the adult should begin with very closed topics and gradually increase the amount of opening as the child does better at closing the utterances with appropriate boundaries.

To teach boundaries, the therapist may use the following approach:

1. Begin with narrow topics such as those suggested by closed questions: "What did you have for lunch?" The response is already present. The adult should also know the answer for the most closed response.
2. Reiterate any utterance made by the child, by imitation or by rephrasing. The child says, "Some chips and a sandwich." The adult then says, "Oh, you had a sandwich and chips for lunch." The child hears what has been said, so additional feedback is provided.
3. Keep the dialogue quickly paced by interrupting verbally so the child can't continue. The rapid pacing will frame the utterance and thus mark the boundaries. For example: "I had, uh a sandwich, and some chips, and, well, I went . . . " "Oh, you had a sandwich and some chips for lunch."

Although most novel utterances by children need to be reinforced for their usage and for the content, the novel utterances of these children are often just rephrases of previously uttered ideas. The following example is taken from a corpora of language that was almost totally devoted to the child trying to talk about the dinosaur: "Ms. Smith, is this a dinosaur?" "Yes, Mary, it is." "Do you think this is really a dinosaur?" "Yes, it is a dinosaur. See how big it is. It is a dinosaur." "Ms. Smith, is this *really* a big dinosaur?" and so forth. The child's novel utterances were really repetitious and should not have been reinforced. The child should have been verbally redirected, as in "Mary, this is a dinosaur, but we were doing our math." When the child does not close a topic, the utterances begin to wander and become off topic, contributing to the topic closure problem.

4. When a question is answered, replace indefinite pronouns with the same words used in the question. For example: "Is this a dinosaur?" "Yes, this is a dinosaur" rather than "Yes, it is." Now the child needs to make the transition from dinosaur to the next idea.

5. If the child is really having problems moving to another idea or topic, ask the child to reiterate the adult's answer. For example: "Is this a dinosaur?" "Yes, this is a dinosaur. What is this?" Notice that the child has been given the question and the answer, which is then followed by the question one more time.

6. If the child has not stopped the rephrasing by now, give him or her the option to say the question or rephrasing one more time. For example, "Mary, I'll answer the question just one more time. This is a dinosaur." Then, if possible, redirect and ignore the topic. Remind the child only once that the answer will be given one more time.

The goals and objectives may not emphasize topic closure work since the purpose of the intervention for this is to replace the closure difficulties with better language skills rather than to increase topic closure. If the clinician or teacher wishes to take data on this problem, the most feasible method is to allow a spontaneous session (without intervention) and determine the percentage of time devoted to rephrasing or showing lack of topic closure, compared to a baseline. Be sure the figure does not include adult shared time. The risk in providing time for spontaneous language is that the activity may facilitate a lack of topic closure. A reduction in topic closure should be accompanied by an increase in effective speech acts.

Sometimes the child isn't simply rephrasing or rambling on without knowing the boundaries. The child's verbalizations may feature new information and new utterances. This indicates that the child has a different semantic language problem, tangentiality.

TANGENTIALITY

Two techniques are best for tangential utterances:

1. Avoid these utterances by narrowing the topic and by keeping the child on target with close-ended questions.

2. *Always* redirect the child so the verbal limits are known. Since normal conversation between two people often involves an occasional tangent, adults often allow children to lead the conversation even if the child is being tangential. But these children tend to lead the conversation to associated ideas or referents, and they need consistent structure and redirection to stay on topic. Never allow these children to stray. Spontaneous activities (those that do not allow the adult to control by models and redirections) are not recommended until the child learns better communication skills.

ECHOLALIA

Researchers have been trying to eliminate echolalia for years. The following techniques, in combination, usually work for most children:

1. Ignore the echolalia if the child has some spontaneous utterances that can be reinforced by allowing the spontaneous utterances to modify or change a hearer's attitudes, beliefs, or behavior. The child's use of the spontaneous utterances supports the social reinforcement of communication while discouraging nonpurposive speech.

2. Use echolalia as the speech act. If the child will echo a model in context, then the child produces an utterance that has the appropriate propositional content. The context assures that the preparatory rule is met for the initial utterance but not for the echoed utterances, the sincerity rule is met by arranging the context, and the child meets the essential elements by the model. So although the imitation cannot be a true speech act, the child's practice in using these rules increases the likelihood that the child will perform a speech act that does meet all the requirements. An example of this method follows: The adult says, "Want some paper." The child echoes, "Want some paper," so the child is given the paper.

3. Produce in a soft voice the parts of questions, pronouns, or anything that cannot be repeated if it is to be appropriate by content. For example, "I (softly) want the paper (louder)." The child's use of "I" would be suggesting or fostering nonintentionally based language.

4. Replace the echolalia with a lower language level that is spontaneous. Many children can echo at a higher level of syntax and morphology than is expected on the basis of their semantic level of development. Return to the semantic level of relations and functions, and then build the language through the techniques previously mentioned.

5. Use an alternate mode to attach referential meaning to the oral-to-aural system and build from the basic semantic level. Alternate modes include sign language, manual communication boards, Bliss symbolics, REBUS reading systems, and so forth. The literature has several reviews of the methods that may be used (Archer, 1977; Dever, 1974; Hollis & Carrier, 1978; Premack & Premack, 1974; Silverman, 1979). The alternate mode is used more as a learning device or supplemental mode than as a separate system for language acquisition.

VERBAL PERSEVERATION

Verbal perseveration can be greatly reduced by alleviating the pressure or stress of the speaking situation. Stress is often created by nonmeaningful tasks, by too high a level of cognitive input, by materials that are too abstract, by pacing that is too fast, by direct questions that use the child's name to signal the child that after being a hearer she or he will be a speaker, and by routines that are broken and consequently change the child's expectations. Therefore, if the materials are at the child's level of thinking, if the routines are maintained, and if the adult uses more comments than direct questions the child's verbal perseveration should be reduced. Daily activities that are comfortable and familiar also provide a starting place for building the environment to include novel ideas and unexpected changes. As most of the literature regarding children or adults with known brain damage suggests, stress can also be eliminated by removing the child or the activity, whichever is easier.

SUMMARY OF THE REMEDIATION TECHNIQUES

The remediation of a child with any of these specific semantic language problems or disorders may include techniques from any or most of the problems since the etiologies and symptoms overlap greatly. However, the educator and clinician need to try to ascertain the language disorder as accurately as the methods allow, because some of the disorders with similar symptoms vary a great deal in reason for existence and therefore need to be treated separately. For example, a child with spatio-temporal difficulties may use many interjections, indicative of the child with word-finding problems. But treatment for word-finding problems will not assist this child. If the problems are difficult to separate, a rule of thumb is that if a treatment doesn't show immediate changes, however minute, then reevaluate the diagnosis as well as the objectives and corresponding methods.

The term *general semantic disorder* has been mentioned several times in this chapter. Most children will exhibit two or more of these problems simultaneously, and this overlap usually indicates that there is some interaction in the breakdown of semantic development. For example, a child who perseverates will usually have some semantic word errors, which often results in semantically based syntax or word order difficulties, which upsets the semantic relationships, and then the child shows some tangentiality or closure difficulties. A breakdown in the child's semantic acquisition results in some overall delay in language development as well as some specific language disorders, thus the term *general semantic disorder*. This term describes patterns of behavior and is not a diagnostic label.

The theoretical basis that underlies the techniques described in this chapter comes from the normal language development literature regarding exceptional children. Although ideally the goal would be for normal progression and systematic intervention, normal development is in fact only a guideline. Many of these children will never be systematic or sequential in their development, and educators must acknowledge this. The techniques are meant to intervene and bypass those aspects of normal development that are preventing the child from acquiring a system of communication that is effective and efficient.

The following principles of remediation are put forth as guidelines in the treatment of semantic disorders:

- Use activities and materials that are in the natural environment, since semantic features or characteristics are needed to build the meaning of the language.

- Use activities that are at the child's basic cognitive level of development, since lexical acquisition depends on the child's internalization about his or her experiences.

- If the form of the language is needed, it should be in the educational plan and not provided by eliminating the meaningful and relevant information of the context.

- Make the language that the child is acquiring function for the child in settings that are as natural as possible. Chapter 8 deals with establishing the natural setting.

These principles should be considered in all objectives, methods, and techniques used to alleviate the different semantic problems. It should also be reemphasized that many of the specific language disorders are eliminated by increasing the positive semantic language development and thus replacing the undesired linguistic skills. However, there are some very specific abilities that can be fostered to enhance semantic development. All clinical intervention and classroom settings should of course encourage the appropriate language usage, since the teachers and clinicians may use many of the techniques throughout the day. The necessary requirement for success would be an appropriate qualitative analysis to determine which skills to encourage and which ones to eliminate. Therefore, the success of intervention depends on the adult's ability to evaluate the child's skills.

The language sample in Table 7-1 was obtained in a free play situation. The six-year-old child took two-and-a-half hours to make the 48 utterances listed on the sample (a period of time considerably longer than expected). Play was used rather than pictures because, even though the child is six years of age, he is very immature socially and functions at a much lower cognitive level than his chronological age would suggest. The materials would usually be more appropriate for a three- or four-year-old child. The utterances on the left of the chart are the child's productions; the adult's utterances are in parentheses. The disorders or symptoms are listed in the middle column, and the remediation is suggested in the right column.

As an inspection of the analysis demonstrates, the child has several problems that overlap. The product of these semantic difficulties is reduced effectiveness in communicating an idea or intent to a hearer in a manner that is represented in conventional form. Chapter 8 discusses the therapeutic methods used with pragmatic problems.

Table 7-1 An Analysis of a Child's Language

Utterance	Symptom	Remediation/Facilitation
1. "What do toys." ("I don't know.")	1. Form and chosen words do not clearly specify intent which was either "What toys shall we play with?" or "What shall we do?" etc.	1. Increase semantic knowledge for specifying referents.
2. "I gonna put fork right here." ("Okay.")	2. Semantic development is fine; the lack of functors is normal development of syntax and morphology but is also key to level of the child's language acquisition.	2. Model appropriate forms.
3. "I put right here." ("Uh, huh.")	3. Recipient or object of action is absent.	3. Semantic referents are missing so knowledge needs to be increased.
4. "That's a big." ("It is?")	4. Child has been in therapy emphasizing vocabulary at the expense of concepts because "big" is not in relationship to its referent.	4. Space/quality remediation for better conceptual knowledge of perceptual and functional attributes.
5. "No big there." ("Where?")	5. Utterance refers to a small as opposed to big object—again, referent is missing.	5. Space/quality remediation.
6. "Small one." ("Small what?")	6. This is actually a label utterance which is an aberrant use of qualifiers as well as an unusual purpose for speaking in this situation.	6. Weakness in semantic basis. Pragmatic emphasis needs to be incorporated into therapy.
7. "Big one." ("Bg what?")	7. Child is not attending to adult's utterances indicating lack of topic identification, probably because of lack of semantic basis as expressed in #6.	7. Same as #3, 4, 5, 6, and add topic identification problems to the list needed to be remediated.
8. "Choo-choo train."	8. Label—primitive function.	8. Semantic basis (relations and functions) to increase pragmatic language.
9. "No big one."	9. Child shows negation in an assertion, but the language doesn't function for further learning nor is it directed at a hearer.	9. Same as previous comments.

(continues)

Table 7-1 continued

Utterance	Symptom	Remediation/Facilitation
10. "This is a small one."	10. Again, the child's previous therapy experiences	10. Same as above. It should be evident
11. "This is a small block."	11. are too obvious. For seven utterances, the language has been nonfunctional, not even egocentric and the utterances, atypical, nonsystematic emergence.	11. that the structural emphasis in therapy is at the expense of the semantic relations and functions missing in the absence of purposive language.
12. "Put this fork in there." ("Okay.")	12. Good purpose and function. The utterance shows intent, referential clarity, and it affects a hearer.	12. ___
13. "Look at fireman." ("Okay.")	13. Same as #12. The lack of functors is developmental.	13. ___
14. "You put that fork in there." ("Okay.")	14. This is a good utterance but keep the context as a consideration. The child goes from #12 (fork) to #13 (fireman) to #14 (fork). Notice the lack of expressing actions or using the toys for play or in a symbolic way.	14. Semantic basis may be lacking as a result of child's inability to focus on the perceptual and functional attributes.
15. "You do ___ too." ("What?")	15. Unintelligible. Probably a phonological neologism or auditory misperception. Child's articulation is too good for it to be an articulatory problem.	15. Verbal correction as they occur and repetition required by child.
16. "I put a block away." ("Those blocks?")	16. Child does not attend to adult's verbalizations. A raise in intensity would be necessary. The child is putting several blocks away, indicating lack of semantic understanding of plural, etc.	16. Semantic concepts.
17. "He's got that chicken." ("What do you mean?")	17. This doesn't make sense in the context. Then child picks up a plastic chicken and fireman. "That" should be "this."	17. Indefinite referential clarity needs verbal redirection and structured activities for encouraging lexical concepts (like those suggested in this chapter for semantic word errors or those in Chapter 6).

18. "Better get that chicken."	18. This is directed to the child who gets the chicken. Ineffective rule order—there's no consequence.	18. Pragmatic therapy.
19. "He is going."	19. Therapy is obvious. So far, the child has worked on size words, "This is ____" and "verbing."	19. Modeling in semantic therapy will improve use of semantic referents and will break up these forms.
20. "Truck."	20. Label.	20.
21. "This is fine truck."	21. Structural expansion of label.	21. Semantic relations and functions needed.
22. "Fireman car." ("Yeh, it's a fire truck.")	22. It's a fire truck. This utterance does show a possessive semantic relation.	22. Same as above.
23. "Fireman truck."	23. Self-correction, but it's not a fire truck.	23. Referents needed.
24. "He's open ____." ("What?")	24. Neologism or auditory misperception.	24. Correct when in error when there's enough semantic basis to understand intention.
25. "He's open number."	25. Child points to the number on the truck. Syntactic error.	25. Result of lack of semantic development.
26. "We look at this." ("You want to look at the book?")	26. Request with command prosody. Child's not attending to the environmental verbal or nonverbal cues. Again the utterances lack referential meaning.	26. Pragmatic therapy.
27. "Puppy chewing." ("Yes.")	27. This refers to the picture and probably is representative of the child's functional linguistic level.	27. For the child's chronological age, the child is severely delayed in the acquisition of basics. This is precipitating the disorders.
28. "Puppy chewing good book." ("Uh, huh.")	28. The child expresses intended agent, object, and action relationship. The "good" is unclear or ambiguous in this content.	28. Lack of referential clarity requires semantic development with materials aimed at a child between 3 and 6.

(continues)

Table 7-1 continued

Utterance	Symptom	Remediation/Facilitation
29. "Puppy chewing the book."	29. The child reevaluates his previous utterance and changes the qualifier. It should be evident that the child's use of structures is inconsistent. Sometimes "the" is omitted before the object and sometimes "is" is included in the present progressive tense. This is definitely not systematic.	29. Increase in referents will improve the child's linguistic ability to formulate his ideas.
30. "Bad little _____."	30. This is said to the picture in the book. Purpose and/or function is naive and is probably another neologism, especially since auditory misperceptions are unrecognizable.	30. Same as previous neologisms and auditory misperceptions.
31. "He's biting ball." ("Yes, the puppy is chewing the ball!")	31. Child needs specific referents and omission of copula is developmental—good expression of semantic relationships.	31. Vocabulary representative of conceptual knowledge.
32. "Cereal." ("What do you want?")	32. This is out of context. There's not enough linguistic skills to express the child's needs or desires.	32. The child lacks an ability to use speech acts; therefore, he needs semantic rule development for pragmatic skills.
33. "I like cereals Dallas." ("Oh, you want the cereal you bought in Dallas.")	33. Dallas is a town and could be a syntactic error. The child was using Dallas as a possessive or it could be part of a prepositional phrase denoting place.	33. Because the preparatory rules are assumed by the child, the hearer isn't ready but tries to meet the child's needs.
34. "Get that."	34. Child grabbed clinician's hand. The use of nonverbal skills illustrates the child's need to assist his linguistic abilities. Adult gets the cereal out of backpack.	34. Semantic/pragmatic remediation.

35. "No open." ("Yep. Cereal's gone.") — The clinician closed the cereal box and put it away. — Semantic relations and functions need to be expanded. Child needs more vocabulary and conceptual information.

36. "Are you open." — This was not a question and a tangential utterance from #35. — Tangentiality techniques.

37. "Now, open a door." ("I don't think so.") — Child is commanding from tangential utterance. — Same as #36.

38. "Take that off." ("What?") — "That" referred to Sheryl—an indefinite term for a person. — Semantic development.

39. "It's a Sheryl." — He responded to the clinician's question, "What," and explained his term "that." Sheryl is the clinician. — This is an unusual usage due to semantic word errors that necessitate techniques for remediation of these.

40. "Ge: that _____." — Again, it was probably a phonological neologism. — Neologism techniques.

41. "Look at that boy." — He's looking at the pictures. Intent is good, utterance has purpose, and message is clear. — ———

42. "You not a girl." ("Yes, I'm a girl.") — Basic problem with concepts; semantic word error. — Activities to decrease semantic word errors.

43. "Now you read that book." ("Okay.") — "That" was used for "this." — Same as #42.

44. "He's chewing." ("Uh, huh.") — Label for picture. — Primitive function necessitates therapy for pragmatic development.

45. "He's chew, uh-oh." — "Uh-oh" is a filler for a referent. — Referential clarity needed through semantic word error activities.

46. "Apples in a tree." — Incomplete proposition—a referent is established but not a full predication. — Semantic relationships need to be expanded.

47. "Sheryl backpack." — Expresses a possessive function in rudimentary form. — More adultlike forms will be facilitated through modeling, while improving semantic basis.

48. "Sheryl give that cereal." — Semantic word errors with intent unclear. The intent could have been better expressed with two words. — He wants the cereal but lacks semantics and thus the morphological skills to express his intent by performing a speech act.

Questions

1. Why does semantic development affect the structural complexity of the child's utterances as well as the overall communicative effectiveness?

2. How does one determine material levels for children with semantic difficulties?

3. Why are some of the semantic symptoms directly remediated while others are assisted through intervention aimed at improving other semantic skills?

4. Why is echolalia so difficult to eliminate without providing some other, more positive form of speaking?

5. How do the various disorders interact?

REFERENCES

Archer, L. A. Blissymbolics—A nonverbal communication system. *Journal of Speech and Hearing Disorders*, 1977, *42*, 568-579.

Brown, R., & Bellugi, U. Three processes in the child's acquisition of syntax. In E. H. Lenneberg (Ed.). *New directions in the study of language*. Cambridge, Mass.: MIT Press, 1964.

Cazden, C. B. *Child language and education*. New York: Holt, Rinehart, & Winston, 1972.

Dever, R. B. Discussion summary—Nonspeech communication. In R. L. Schiefelbusch and L. L. Lloyd (Eds.), *Language perspectives, acquisition, and retardation*. Baltimore, Md.: University Park Press, 1974.

Hollis, J. H., & Carrier, J. K. Intervention strategies for nonspeech children. In R. L. Schiefelbusch (Ed.), *Language intervention strategies*. Baltimore, Md.: University Park Press, 1978.

Lee, L. *Interactive language development teaching*. Evanston, Ill.: Northwestern University Press, 1975.

Lucas, E. V. The feasibility of speech acts as a language approach for emotionally disturbed children. (Doctoral dissertation, University of Georgia, 1977). *Dissertation Abstracts International*, 1978, *38*, 3479B-3967B. (University Microfilms No. 77-30, 488).

McLean, J., & Snyder-McLean, L. *A transactional approach to early language training*. Columbus, Ohio: Charles E. Merrill, 1978.

Muma, J. R. Language intervention: Ten techniques. *Acta Symbolica*, 1970, *1*, 43-46.

Mundell, C., & Lucas, E. *A parent conducted pragmatic language program for Down's Syndrome children*. An unpublished manuscript, Washington State University, 1978.

Premack, D., & Premack, A. J. Teaching visual language to apes and language deficient persons. In R. L. Schiefelbusch & L. L. Lloyd (Eds.), *Language perspectives, acquisition, and retardation*. Baltimore, Md.: University Park Press, 1974.

Rebus Materials. Salt Lake City, Utah: Word Making Productions, 1973.

Silverman, F. *Communication for the speechless*. New York: Prentice-Hall, 1979.

CHAPTER OBJECTIVES

- plan a session for facilitating pragmatic language skills.

- explain the purpose, rationale, methods, and anticipated implementation of this approach to parents and colleagues.

- carry out a therapy session for pragmatic language facilitation.

- explain methods for providing contexts and opportunities for speech acts.

- take data on speech act performances for therapy accountability.

- write the goals and objectives for facilitating speech acts in language disordered children.

- explain the relationship between semantic development and speech act performance.

- explain the principles of the speech act and how these principles relate to therapy development.

- explain the results obtained from a therapy approach that are aimed at facilitating the performance of speech acts.

- describe the types of speech acts most frequently used by young children and the relationship of these speech acts to the child's environment.

Chapter 8

A Remediation Procedure for Pragmatic Language Disorders

Expectations are a self-fulfilling
prophecy of any given communication dyad.

Pragmatic language refers to the speaker's use of linguistic and paralinguistic skills to convey a proposition intended to alter a hearer's attitudes, beliefs, or behaviors. The pragmatic unit of analysis chosen for use in this book is the speech act as described by the semantic rules outlined in Chapter 2. The previous chapters have examined those disorders that result from problems with the components governed by the semantic rules. This chapter attempts to facilitate the semantic rules as part of a gestalt speech act. Whenever the components are deficient, incomplete, altered, or deviant, the effectiveness of the speaker's message is reduced. If a child's verbalizations are effective in attempting to alter the hearer's attitudes, beliefs, or behaviors, then the child has performed a speech act. If a child is not effective or does not attempt to convey intent through the conventional linguistic skills, then the child is not performing speech acts even though the attempts to try are evident. This chapter will present methods for facilitating speech act performance.

PREREQUISITES FOR PERFORMING SPEECH ACTS

To be an effective performer of speech acts, the child needs to have a conventional set of symbols, a hearer, and a context. In a spoken language community the conventional set of symbols is the sound system (speech) aided by nonverbal gestures, body movements, and cues. Alternate modes (such as signed language or manual communication) may constitute the conventional set of symbols in some communities. A hearer is a necessary prerequisite since the absence of a hearer makes it impossible for the speaker to alter another's attitudes, beliefs or behaviors. The conventional set of symbols and the hearer become part of the context. The context includes all the preconceived knowledge about the situation that is shared by the speaker and the hearer as well as the nonlinguistic features of the environment. Within this context, the child has the opportunity to perform a speech act. The incorporation of any given speech act into the entire context is accomplished by the performance of a speech event. The speech event changes when the basic constituents of the context are modified. The types of speech acts may continue to be performed even though the speech event is different. For the purposes of clinical or educational intervention, this chapter will concentrate on facilitating the performance of speech acts. The semantic disorders outlined and discussed in previous chapters are more likely to affect the speech event.

The ideal setting for facilitating a child's performance of speech acts is one in which the child can use language to convey intentions in ways that can affect the hearer immediately. When the hearer is affected in a way the child can observe, this satisfies the child's needs and acts as an immediate reinforcement. The speech acts used most often by children with language development below five years of age include requests for objects, requests for action, requests for information, summons or callings, rule orderings, denials (rejections, etc), assertions, and statements of information. These speech acts are based on literature in normal development (Bates, 1976; Dore, 1973; Bruner, 1974) as well as on clinical application (Brown, 1979; Hoag, 1975; Lucas, 1977; Mundell & Lucas, 1978). The following strategy for facilitating pragmatic language is aimed at teaching a child to perform the most common speech acts.

Since the child meets daily needs by performing speech acts, the child's teacher or parent will want to examine some of the ways the child could use language. The following list assumes that the representative utterances are in context and meet the rules for speech acts. The assumption is an important consideration, since any one utterance may be governed by different semantic rules and thus convey a different intent. For example, if a child requests a piece of paper, the child might say, "Give me the paper." But in a different setting the child might say, "Give me the paper?" indicating a request for information as to whether the child should have the paper. The following list suggests the variety of utterances that might be used to express specific speech acts. Examples (Lucas, 1977) of the eight common speech acts as found in young children are provided below:

Speech Act	Context
1. Requests for objects	The child knows that someone has an object that he or she wants. The child requests the object.

Examples include:	"Want cookie," "May I have a cookie?" "Gimme the glue."
2. Requests for actions	The child believes that he needs the action of another child or adult is needed.
Examples include:	"Go away." "Me up" (pick me up), "Would you please pour the juice?" "Help me." "Tie my shoe."
3. Assertions	The child says something that he believes to be true. He does not think that the listener knows this.
Examples include:	"That doggie," "No, it's a car." "That's the biggest horse ever." "Daddy's car."
4. Denials	The hearer or someone in the context does something that the child does not accept. The child believes that the hearer must be told of this action to keep the action from continuing or from occurring again.
Examples include:	"I don't wanna," "no dirty" (to indicate that he doesn't want to wash), "no juice" (to indicate that the child doesn't want the juice put in front).
5. Requests for information	The child feels additional information about the context is needed.
Examples include:	"Time go?" "Daddy home?" "Why do birds die?" "How come we got to go to school?" "Where's Jimmy?"
6. Callings	The child wants to call attention to the next utterance or to the immediate area or to simply gain another's attention.
Examples include:	"Morning," "Hey you," "Yoo-hoo," "Look," "Sue."
7. Stating information	The child has something to tell that is not common knowledge to the speaker and hearer. The only way the hearer would know this is by the child telling the hearer.
Examples include:	"Mommy bakes cookies." "I found a dollar bill." "My brother is a meany." "I found my dog."
8. Rule ordering	The child believes that something needs to be told to the hearer to change the actions of that person.

Examples include: "You're not 'spoze' to play with matches."
"Stop pulling the swing." "Let go of my bi-
cycle." (indicates that the rule is that no one
else plays with his bicycle), "Mine."

All of the speech act examples cited above were part of a context so that the child is attempting to convey an intent to a hearer. In these examples the child has contextual referents to use and a setting in which the needs may be met. As described in Chapter 2, the speech act is based on four principles: linguistic behavior (1) is rule governed, (2) is part of an active process, (3) is the expression of a speaker's intent, and (4) is an integral part of a communication process. Each of these principles should be considered in developing the context and meeting other requirements of the intervention setting. As one of the speech act components, the context must have activity so that there are ways to change behavior. Clinically the activity must be free of adult domination so the child has the time and place to practice talking about the activity.

Most classrooms and homes can function as excellent contexts in which a child can use language in a variety of ways. The sterile therapy room is not a good site for conversational exchange.

The remediation suggestions in this chapter are based on research in which classroom teachers and aides in special education were taught to facilitate language in a class that consisted of six to eight special needs school-age children (Lucas, 1977), and also on research in which parents were taught to use the same techniques at home with Down's Syndrome infants (Mundell & Lucas, 1978). The suggestions have been shared with public school classroom teachers and preschool teachers for the handicapped and nonhandicapped. Those who have implemented the techniques have expressed satisfaction with the good to excellent results. Furthermore, the data from this research (Lucas, 1977; Lucas & Mundell, 1978) suggest that facilitating language usage greatly increases the child's syntax, morphology, and frequency of production. Therefore, the small amount of effort devoted to the training of parents, classroom teachers, and clinicians is well worth the trainee's and trainer's time.

Once a context has been determined, the adult must be willing to exchange speaker-hearer roles with the child. A child can be effective in performing speech acts only if the child can affect a hearer. If a child is being asked to respond in expected ways, then the child is not intentionally influencing a hearer. To influence the hearer, the child must produce a spontaneous utterance within a given context and to which a hearer may respond. The adult must realize that this exchange of speaker and hearer roles makes it possible for the adult to act as a speaker as well as a responder.

Given a context and an awareness that the role exchange is required for production of a speech act, the child is given positive chances to use speech and body aspects to affect the hearers (adults and children) in the environment. These chances are provided through tasks that allow the child to speak and change the context accordingly. The procedure used for implementing this system is as simple as the underlying basis: *Provide the child with the tools and the opportunity to be a successful communicator, and the child has been given the purpose to maintain lingustic communication.* The procedure has been outlined in the following sections of this chapter.

DETERMINING THE APPROPRIATE INTERVENTION

Not all language disordered children need to be enrolled in a program emphasizing language usage. If the child has difficulty using the linguistic process for communication, then the child's problem necessitates a program that emphasizes learning how to use linguistic skills. This rationale is based on the theoretical notion that children won't acquire language skills they don't use, and that using language skills generates more language.

The children who should be put into this type of program may be identified by behavioral observations, anecdotal records, and/or by a criterion referenced measure such as the BISAP. (These identification procedures were described in Chapter 6.) There is one other identification consideration: When do a child's semantic disorders affect language usage, requiring a shift in emphasis away from remediation of the disorders to emphasizing better language usage?

The semantic language disorders described in Chapter 3 do affect communication effectiveness, and theoretically this is expected since the speech act is governed by the semantic constituent rules. If the semantic rules are impinged on, then the child's intended message is affected. The overall negative effects must be weighed against the child's needs. For example, does the child need to learn how to request, or does the child need to learn to stay on topic so that the requesting is effective? This basic assessment can be made after a language sample is obtained and qualitatively analyzed, after anecdotal records about the child's behavior are examined, and after a measure such as the BISAP is used.

If the child's semantic disorders, while affecting message conveyance, are not destroying the pragmatic process, then the BISAP need not be administered and intervention for the specific problems may proceed. If the child is manipulating the environment physically and nonverbally or passively responding to it verbally or nonverbally, then the child is not attempting speech acts and should be considered a candidate for intervention to improve language usage (prior to working directly on the semantic disorders). The criterion for the semantic or pragmatic emphasis is whether or not the child is attempting to perform speech acts. *If the child tries to perform speech acts but the hearer has difficulty following the intended message, then the child needs the semantic emphasis. If the child seldom tries to perform speech acts (usually because the child is a re-*

sponder), then the child needs the pragmatic emphasis or the context for speech act performance.

CONTEXTS

The following section is intended to suggest different types of contexts that tend to provide opportunities for facilitating one or more specific types of speech acts. Other speech acts may be used in each of these contexts, but some situations are predominated by a certain type of speech acts. Therefore, for facilitation, use the context that provides the greatest opportunity for the speech act being fostered.

Requests for Objects

This context suggests that there are some objects that the child wants and that the adult is more than willing to provide these if the child performs or attempts to perform a speech act in accordance with the child's level of development. The means to facilitate the speech acts will be discussed in a later section. The materials and activities that have proven to be the most effective for requests for objects include art tasks, snack or meal times, work tasks, clothing or dressing times, and hygiene tasks. The objects include art materials, work materials, clothing articles, and objects for hygiene.

Requests for Actions

If physical assistance is needed during work or play, the child should request that the adult assist. Help during the mealtime or during dressing also requires a request for action.

Assertions

Assertions (either a positive or negative utterance) may be facilitated during or after art tasks. The assertion is usually facilitated by asking the child to talk or tell about the finished or partly completed tasks. This type of asserting may be facilitated for the adult as the hearer or for the other children as hearers. The assertion may also be facilitated before or after story times or activity experiences. The assertion requires that the speaker and the hearer have both participated in the task. The child wants to let the hearer know that the child also knows the idea being asserted. If the hearer weren't familiar with the information, then the utterance would probably be a statement of information.

Denials

Denials—which include rejection of objects, actions, and/or events—may be facilitated by giving or doing to the child something opposite or different from what the child had requested during work, play, meal, and/or art time.

Requests for Information

These requests may be facilitated during an activity in which some essential information has been deleted, so that the child must request information in order to complete the task. Academic and art tasks and new games are good contexts for facilitating this type of speech act. The context must provide some novel or unfamiliar aspect that the child does not know or cannot solve without asking for information. Any activity that is new to a child will provide this type of context.

Callings or Summons

This context is facilitated whenever the presence of an adult or child is necessary in an activity. This is particularly true when another person is needed for a game, when the person being called has something the child needs, or when the child needs someone to come and assist in an activity. The assistance may be needed on the playground, in the cafeteria, or in the classroom. The important feature of these contexts is that the hearer—the person being called—must be at a reasonable distance from the child to necessitate the calling.

Stating Information

To state information, the content or proposition must be unknown to the hearer. The best contexts are those that provide an opportunity to talk about home activity while at school or about school activity while at home. Some good contexts include share time situations, news events, or discussions about a child's activities during school or after school.

Rule Ordering

While acquiring language, the child also acquires an understanding of the rules that govern school and home environments. Rule orders are facilitated in any setting in which the child can tell someone else the rules. Play and work situations are usually best.

OPPORTUNITY

After the adult has determined the type of contexts available and the variety of utterances that might occur in those contexts, it is important to give the child many opportunities to perform the speech act. The acquisition of the semantic rules that govern speech acts begins in the social exchange between caretaker and infant. Semantic development continues as the child matures, so that the child eventually has a refined and sophisticated linguistic system that enables the speaker to communicate with flexibility and power. It should be noted that this natural process of acquisition often does not occur in the language delayed and/or language disordered child.

How do language disordered children function, linguistically, in simple contexts without direct intervention? The following behavioral observations have been collected from different types of settings, classes, geographic locations, and grade or special grade levels. In any given work or art task, the child with a pragmatic language disorder will wait to be given materials, wait to be told what to do, wait to be asked what he or she is doing, wait to be told to change activities or that he or she is changing the attitudes, beliefs, or behaviors of others in an unconventional way.

For example, a teacher of a preschool class for the handicapped brought a coconut to school and put it in the science area. With the exception of one Down's Syndrome child, all the children were in the class because of language delays or disorders as diagnosed by the school speech and language clinicians. After the coconut had been in the science area for two days, the teacher asked one of the children to go back to the area and see if there was something new. The child went back and looked. He came back to the teacher and reported that he had seen that thing there but didn't know what it was. She told the child to bring it to her. The child brought it and none of the children asked what it was, what it was for, or made any other verbalization. The teacher was amazed! She had taught regular kindergarten and preschool classes for twenty years. She said that in her regular preschool classes the children would have asked about the coconut immediately and their questions would have been incessant. Here in the language disordered children there was a total lack of spontaneous, curious language. Although differences in socioeconomic or cultural backgrounds may sometimes explain differences in asking behavior, these variables were not operating in this situation; here the only difference was the language disorders. This example of a discrepancy between spontaneous, curious language used to further linguistic development and the language disordered child's inflexibility may help explain the plateau of other linguistic skills in the language disordered child.

When language disordered children are asked to go and do a task, they will often wait to be asked at the other end about their presence. For example, if a teacher tells a language disordered child to go sharpen pencils in the office, the child will go to the office but once there will wait for the secretary to ask what the child wants. The secretary's desire to help the child is a function of the societal speech act rules: A speaker does not turn and signal the readiness of an utterance without following through.

The pragmatically disordered children seldom attempt to buy their own items in a store, but neither do they ask to do it. If two children get into a fight on the playground, the fight is going to be physical and not verbal unless it's automatic and is verbally abusive. Then everyone who gets in the child's way also receives the verbal onslaught, indicating a lack of intention or purpose for the verbal remarks. If the language disordered child needs help with a task or with following directions, he or she will mess up the task, not do it, or "act out" in order to get the attention. If the language disordered child needs to go to the bathroom, he or she will get the teacher's attention physically or walk out of the classroom. Although some of these children are inappropriate tattletales, it is unlikely that they will report an event that is needed to carry out the normal routine. For example, recall the previous description of the adolescent who watched the washing machine overflow but was not interested or was not expected to report this information.

This implies that the adolescent may have reported the event had she been expected to report. Yes! The opportunity to perform speech acts implies the expectation of the hearer as part of the preparatory rule. The preparatory rule is designed to include both the speaker and the hearer in the context. For example, in a request for an object, the context includes the speaker who wants the object *and* a hearer who can give the object. The speaker won't ask for the object unless it is obvious to the speaker that the hearer is in a position to give the object. The expectation of the hearer, then, is a critical element of context— more specifically, a critical element of the preparatory rule. Without the expectation being satisfied, the hearer and the speaker will not engage in conversation; the basic rules for the performance of the speech act are incomplete. Since the preparatory aspect occurs before the utterance, the speaker won't even attempt to perform a speech act unless the preparatory rule has been met.

In the example of the overflowing washing machine, it took several minutes to convince the adolescent that reporting the incident would have been a good and appropriate thing to do. This was because when the adolescent went to tell the staff members about the incident, one staff member said, "And why are you telling me?" The adolescent turned to the accompanying adult as if to say, "I told you so." The adult told the staff member why the incident was being reported: "I thought you might want to stop the machine, maybe clean up the mess, etc." At this point the staff member sought help. The expectation dyad worked two ways. The staff member didn't expect the adolescent to be reporting anything of significance since much of her talking was nonfunctional—that is, her language really did not affect the hearer in any significant or observable way.

It is difficult to determine the point at which the child and the significant people no longer assume language to be effective at communicating. This breakdown usually begins early in the preschool years. The children do not expect to be hearers, and, in many instances, the adults do not expect the children to be speakers. Most adults who have worked with special education children, even at the preschool level, soon lower their expectations. Not all teachers of the handicapped are like the teacher with the coconut. She did expect the children to talk, and when they didn't talk, she intervened.

This chapter is intended to instigate the child's participation as a speaker and the adult's participation as a hearer. If the context is suitable and the preparatory rules are not violated, then the child should want to express a proposition with the sincere desire to affect the hearer—provided that the hearer is able to discern the child's attempt at the essential components of the speech act.

The adult's or facilitator's role in the context is to first provide the opportunity and then direct the child through the necessary steps for successful performances of various speech acts by providing the child with prompts, models, and cues. There are several ways (verbal and nonverbal) to create the opportunity.

Opportunities to use language or to perform a speech act may start with the adult producing an open utterance, such as:

"Who wants to help?"
"Who can tell me?"
"Want juice, Jimmy?"
"What do you want?"
"Get Mike to play with us."
"Who wants to play the guitar?"
"I have a drum. (pause) Anyone want to see it?"
"What's the matter? Your bike is upside down?"
"Look. Your sleeve is wrong side out."

These types of utterances leave it open for the child to respond verbally (or in some instances nonverbally) to the adult. Once the child performs, then the adult has several options. However, the child also has several choices as to how and whether to respond.

Opportunities may also be provided by placing materials in the child's visual field or by introducing a task. The context should provide verbal and nonverbal signals that encourage the child to respond linguistically. But what if the child responds verbally but says something that does not fit the context or does not complete the essential components of the speech act. The child who does not respond or who responds inappropriately needs a model.

Models

Since the semantic rules of the speech act are part of the social skills as well as part of the linguistic skills, the child needs both the social and linguistic model to imitate. Therefore, the only acceptable social and linguistic model is another person performing the speech act. This other person can't be the facilitator. If the facilitator models the speech act, then the sincerity and preparatory rules are violated; the child doesn't have any purpose for performing the speech act because the hearer (the facilitator) already knows what the child wants.

The model could be a peer who is language delayed but doesn't experience any basic problems with pragmatic skills, a non-language-delayed or non-language-disordered peer, a sibling, or another adult such as an aide or parent. For example, if a teacher takes a xylophone from the closet, the child with normal language development will comment or ask about the instrument: "Are we having music today?" "Can I play it?" "What are we going to do?" The language disordered child would probably ignore the xylophone. If the model makes a comment like, "Let me play it, please," then the disordered child has the opportunity to follow the model's lead. The model shows the child what visual and auditory behaviors are expected for that situation, increasing the likelihood that the child will perform a speech act in the same preparatory situation in this context or in any other similar context governed by the same rules. The materials, in this instance the xylophone, don't really make a difference; it's the preparatory rules that are the same.

Examples of open utterances that provide opportunities for speech acts are listed below. In these contexts, the language disordered child did not respond, so the model responded.

Adult or Parent	*Model*
"Who wants help?"	"I do. I want help."
"Who can tell me?"	"I can. I see a bird."
"Want juice, Jimmy?"	"Yes, give me some."
"What do you want?"	"Gimme a fork."
	"Paper."
	"Glue, please, or paper."
"Get Mike to play."	"Mike. Come on. Play."
"Who wants to play the guitar?"	"I do. I'll play."
"I have a drum." (pause)	"I want to see it."
"What's the matter? Your bike is upside down."	"Help. Help my bike."
"Your sleeve is wrong side out."	"Here."

Variety of Models

Notice the variety of utterances in the previous examples. It is important that the person who is modeling the speech act provide a variety of constructions or productions. The greater the variety, the better the chance the child will learn the underlying semantic rules rather than the specific constructions. The following principles must be considered when providing the child with an opportunity and a model.

1. Always vary the utterance form. If requests for objects are the desired type of speech act, then use a variety of forms, such as "Gimme the X," "I want the X," "Can I have the X," "Pass the X," "Let me have the X," etc. By not varying the utterance forms, the child learns the construction (such as "I want X") but not the semantic rules.
2. Vary the contexts when facilitating a single type of speech act, such as requests for objects. If the purpose is to increase the functional language, then the child needs many contexts in which to practice making these requests. If snack time is the only context used, then the child has learned a task-specific skill and not the underlying semantic rules.
3. The model provides a linguistic example as well as a social example. In this way the child can observe the real purpose of the language. Therefore, the model's language level must be commensurate or slightly above the child's syntax and morphology level.

Linguistic Direction

A context has been established, the speech act for facilitation has been determined, the opportunity has been given, and a peer or adult model has been provided when the child does not respond. For some children, this model is still not enough. The child may need practice in direct linguistic imitation to have an experience at changing the hearer and/or the context. The model should reduce the complexity of the utterance to the disordered child's spontaneous linguistic level. For some children, this will be as low as one word. The child needs to produce only one word to perform a rudimentary or primitive speech act and two words (one for referring and one for predicating) to produce an adult speech act. The linguistic expression, of course, as well as the variety of speech acts continues to improve throughout adulthood.

The model, then, provides an utterance at the child's grammatical level or slightly above. If the child doesn't need a direct imitation step, then the adult's utterances should be simple but grammatical. If the child needs this step, then the simple but grammatical utterances should be interspersed with utterances at the child's spontaneous level of production. This is not the child's level of imitation or drill, or echolalia; it is the level at which the child's utterances function to manipulate the environment. The need for input at the child's level indicates the advantage of using peer or sibling models over some adult models who have difficulty speaking like a child.

Direct Cues or Prompts

The child is in a context and has been given the opportunity to perform a speech act, first by an open utterance and then, if necessary, by a model at the child's level of linguistic competence. Now the child is given the open utterance a second time, for another opportunity to perform the speech act. Unfortunately, some children still do not respond linguistically. These children may need a direct cue. The direct cue is the first direct intervention technique. The other components are all part of a natural situation (except for an adult who is acting like a child). The context is naturally providing the opportunity to interact linguistically and obtain the desired effects. The direct cue is a method of telling the child that the facilitator-adult knows the semantic rules that affect the performances of the speech act. The direct cue provides several types of information to the child:

1. The direct cue tells the child about the preparatory or propositional items. For example, in a request for an object, the child wants the object. Most non-language-disordered children assume that the adult can get the object, or the child doesn't ask. The object of the request should be made visible so the child has at least that much information. The adult provides the opportunity with an open utterance such as "Who wants the ball at recess?" (In normal classrooms the children wouldn't have waited for the teacher to ask this question. After the first recess and with the ball in sight, the children would ask the teacher at every recess period before the teacher could say anything.) The teacher has provided a linguistic direction and the model responds. (This is the advantage of having an adult, someone who will wait to see if the language disordered child will perform.) Suppose the child doesn't follow the model by imitation. Now the adult gives the child the preparatory or propositional rules as a direct cue. For example, "Homer, I have a ball." If this utterance, another opportunity, doesn't prompt the child, then another rule is given. A propositional portion of the rules was given, so now the teacher or adult gives the preparatory component: "If you want the ball for recess, you may get it from me." Finally, if the other two direct cues fail, the child is told what to do to get the ball: "Homer ask me for the ball." The following examples are illustrations of direct cues:

Adult	*Adult's Direct Cues*
"What do you want?" (pause)	"Here's the juice."
	"I have a fork."
	"Here's the paper."
"Who wants to play the guitar?" (pause)	"I want to play the guitar."
	"I can help you."
"Your sleeve is wrong side out." (pause)	"I know. (pause) I can help
"Your bike is upside down." (pause)	you."

After the direct cue, the adult looks at the child as if expecting a verbalization.

2. The direct cue provides the child with additional opportunities to perform a speech act that will affect the hearer in this intervention setting. The consequences of this performance (such as obtaining the ball) will act as a reinforcement.

3. The direct cues provide additional semantic information, often in linguistic form, about the perceptual and functional attributes of the situation or events. The child is learning about the environment through the adult's or model's information.

4. The direct cues provide a bridge between the socialization of language (consequences and purposes) and the actual production of linguistic skills.

5. The direct cues provide more linguistic information at the child's level of structural complexity. This input will benefit the child's syntax and morphological development.

Utterance Act Imitation

Even though the direct cues have been given so that everything is available for the child—the context, the opportunities, the rules of the situation, and modeled consequences—some children will need one more step: actual direct manipulation of the child's performance of the utterance act. This usually takes the form of assisting the child in the imitation.

The following examples are provided to illustrate the manner in which this pragmatic process occurs.

1. "Get Garrett to play with us." (no response)
   "I have the ball. Garrett knows how to play." (direct cue)
   "Say: "Garrett play ball." (modeled at child's level)
2. "What do you want?" (no response)
   "Ask me: I want juice." (no response)
   "Say: Give me juice." (at child's level)

3. (A child is struggling with her jacket.)
   "Do you need some help?" (no response—pause)
   "I can help you with your jacket." (direct cue)
   "Ask me for help." (no response)
   "Say: Help me." (at child's level of structural complexity)

These three examples demonstrate how to go from open opportunity, to direct cues (multiple opportunities), to the final direct imitation. If the child doesn't imitate even when told to imitate, then the child does not obtain the consequence and the procedure continues. Each time another child receives a consequence through linguistic means, another model and another opportunity has been provided for the language disordered child.

Suppose a child says, "Want." It is really important that the child obtains the consequences only when she attempts or performs a speech act, even if it is by direct imitation. If the child who doesn't ask continues to obtain what the others are receiving, then that child learns there is no need to perform the speech act.

Pacing

It's critical that the facilitator not directly assist the child with the imitation unless absolutely necessary. It is preferable to use direct cues (semantic rules) so that the child realizes that the environment provides a model. If the child's frustration level is low, then there may be a need to increase the direct imitation prompts. By proceeding at a quick pace through the questions to the answers or consequences, the child's anxiety may be reduced and the number of direct cues increased. The child should be allowed to participate and/or be assisted whenever he or she tries, even though the components of the speech act are not fulfilled. As the number of attempts increases, then the direct models and cues are faded.

Reducing the Cues and Models

Research to date has shown the child with a pragmatic language disorder requires only a few days of direct cues before the cues can be eliminated. Subsequently, even the linguistic models can be omitted. The child will still need to have the linguistic utterances expanded and improved upon and will need a wide variety of experiences or contexts for further learning, but the semantic rules are learned expediently.

There is one condition, however, that must be met if this treatment method is to work: The process must be done with total effort and interest, the techniques and procedures followed consistently and without exceptions. The parents and teachers who are conscious of the techniques throughout the day have better results than those who only *occasionally* use the techniques. Consistent use of the techniques for three or four weeks may produce results, whereas *occasional* use of the techniques over a period of several months may not produce any results.

A logical explanation for the excellent results through consistent techniques is that the child is acquiring a semantic rule system governing the speech act. In order for the child to understand the pattern of the rules, there cannot be any exceptions or deviations that would confuse the rule learning.

Once the rules are acquired, the cues can be removed. An example of the procedure used to fade the cues is presented below:

> "What do you want for drawing your picture?" (no response)
> "I have crayons and pencils." (direct cues—no response)
> "If you want a crayon or pencil, ask me." (direct cues—no response)
> "Say: Red crayon, please."

Later the same morning the child is in a similar setting:

> "Arnold, which one do you want?" (points to crayons and pencils)
> "I have the crayons and pencils." (direct cues—no response)
> "Ask me."
> "Red crayon." (child's response)

The same setting, but later:

> "I still have the crayons and pencils."
> "Pencil." (child responds)
> "You want a pencil, okay." (the adult expands the child's utterances since the child did ask, but the utterance was linguistically incomplete for the question asked)

For the last picture, the materials are still present:

> "We're going to do one more picture." (pause)
> "Ms. Smith, I want some of that paper, please." (peer model)
> "Okay, who else?"
> "I do."
> "Arnold?"
> "Paper." (child responds)

Results

Some of the results of this kind of approach have been unexpected. It was expected that the number and frequency of various speech acts would increase, and they did. It was not expected that the child's syntax and morphology skills would become more complex, but they did. From other reports, the same type of result is being obtained. There is a simple theoretical explanation for the expected and unexpected results.

The child does have multiple opportunities to perform speech acts, which does increase the skills to do this activity. Because the model uses language at or slightly above the child's syntactic and morphological complexity, the child's imitated utterance act has purpose and therefore is also learned. As the model expands on the child's linguistic complexity, the child's linguistic complexity increases.

These results raise some questions regarding language intervention format and rationale. Although syntax and morphology may be drilled effectively and efficiently in second language or dialectical learners, the social purpose coupled with the semantic basis have greater influence over the child's language acquisition. Therefore a program that emphasizes linguistic content and function may be more efficient at facilitating later developing forms. Research will eventually support or reject this hypothesis; but, in the interim, the emphasis on semantic development and language function in the language disordered child is warranted.

ACTIVITIES FOR SPEECH ACTS

The key to establishing an environment for providing speech act opportunities is to make as many problems as possible for the child to solve verbally. The adult becomes a saboteur rather than a doer for the child. As a saboteur, the adult changes the nice, organized environment into one that needs constant verbal interaction. Only possible verbal solutions provide pleasant consequences. The following items and events suggest ways to develop an environment of problems that need verbal solution: taped together scissors, plugged glue bottles, empty or dried-up pens, broken pencil leads, coat sleeves turned inside-out by the morning aide when the children aren't watching, not enough chairs, not enough snacks, cups with holes in the bottom, missing toys, flat balls, short jump ropes, missing colors or paints, not enough paper, no tacks for hanging pictures, tables with missing legs, water faucets turned off tightly, baseballs without bats or bats without baseballs, etc. The problem-solving tasks require more than the performance of speech acts; the tasks necessitate better attending to the environmental cues and thus more discrimination and sorting of the features that lead to knowledge development.

In addition to being a saboteur, the adult must expect the children to get their own coats and their own materials, to share their work with other children, to tell about their finished products, to display their products on their own, to report about events, and so forth. It's easier for parents and other adults to perform most of the child's necessary tasks rather than wait for a child who is slow and who functions at a low verbal level. In one case, a child who had been in the pragmatic therapy setting for a few weeks was taken to an ice cream parlor. The child ordered his own cone, paid for the cone, and ate the cone while sitting at the table. The child also asked if he could go get a drink of water and if he could leave. The process was time consuming but well worth the effort. The following Sunday the child was in the same place with his parent. The parent was in a hurry, and neither the child nor the parent saw the researcher observing. The child flew around the store as if he were an airplane, while the parent did all of the tasks. The child was taken outside to eat the cone because he was embarrassing to the parent. The extra time to establish an environment for the child to be a speaker is well worth the results.

Parent Interveners

Since the pragmatic intervention process is quite simple, the child's parents are capable of learning the techniques and being effective at using them within two or three hour-long sessions. There are some mitigating forces: (1) the parent needs feedback by the trainer between sessions; (2) the parent needs examples from their own home to illustrate the possible opportunities; (3) the parent needs examples of models and direct cues for their specific child; and (4) the parent needs reinforcement for trying. Of course, since the child's progress is usually evident, the parent is reinforced immediately by the results.

Success really depends on the parent's consistent use of the techniques. At the beginning, this type of approach can seem quite complicated. This training period does take time, and the time isn't always available. But once the process is learned, it becomes a simple and natural part of parent-child interaction with the child requiring no additional time except for the time the child needs to perform the speech acts.

Reinforcement

This pragmatic intervention approach suggests that the consequences of a child's linguistic behavior are immediate and their presence increases the likelihood that the child will use speech to obtain desired effects. Certainly the effects do reinforce the child, but it has also been noted that the child's opportunity to *conform, fit in,* and *become one of the others* through participation is another powerful incentive or reinforcer.

Part of the evidence for a reinforcer comes from work with children whose undesirable or negative behaviors cannot be replaced by language through any primary (water, food, sleep) or typical secondary reinforcers (vibration, movement, play, socialization). Although the children's biting, kicking, pulling hair, etc., may be temporarily suppressed (for good attending behavior and responses to verbal and nonverbal tasks), the long-term effects are negligible. In other words, the child does not communicate as an initiator of requests, assertions, denials, rule orders, and so forth.

However, these low-functioning children will communicate at a minimal level if expected to participate. (It is assumed that the child has been assessed nonverbally to determine whether the child has the cognitive ability for the verbal participation.) Again, the model in the intervention setting is allowed to participate, but the language disordered child does not get a chance to participate until a verbal attempt is made. Visual semantic cues supplied by augmenting or supplemental modes such as sign language are suggested so as to provide a visual to auditory association. The minimally verbal child may or may not be expected to participate while using the alternative verbal system.

Entertaining variables depress participation and therefore have to be eliminated. For example, once the model has obtained the paper or objects, the model does the drawing behind a board or divider so the child can't see the activity or the materials. Withholding the sharing of the task provides the opportunity for more speech act facilitation. For example, "Natalie, want to see?"

For a very young or verbally low-functioning child, the constant changing of the tasks provides an additional novelty that also increases the chance that the child will verbalize in a purposive manner. Even for older children, it is important to withhold participation until the speech act attempt is made after direct cues or imitation. If a child can observe the other children and enjoys the spectator role, then the child has no need or purpose for joining the activity. Sometimes it is a good idea to select a removable context, such as a box. For example: "Mary (model) has a box (direct cue) with rabbits in it (could use cars, toys, etc.). Who wants to see the rabbits?" Mary says, "I do. I want to look." Mary opens the lid and looks, "Who else wants to see?" If there's a group of children, there will be takers. If two adults are working with one severely language disordered child, then playing with the rabbits (or cars or whatever) has to occur *in* the box so that the nonverbal child makes a verbal attempt to participate.

Once the child makes a verbal attempt (if this takes time, consider providing an alternate mode rather than the vocal), then the chance to participate must be avoided and immediately removed to increase the number of opportunities for verbal attempts. The most difficult children work to participate in these activities even though they may not work for primary or typical secondary reinforcers. This is possibly an indication of the importance of social interaction in teaching linguistic communication.

There is also evidence that participation is important for compliant children. The evidence lies with the out-of-context results that indicate that the children who learn to perform speech acts are learning rules that govern other situations so that the children use these skills in novel contexts. It is the participation that makes the difference, because a speech act is an active process that has purpose in communication. Theoretically and clinically, any other paradigm that does not include participation would be excluding a principle that would not allow for acquisition of the semantic rules governing the speech act. The child would learn verbal tasks and other components of language but would not learn linguistic behavior as a rule-governed, purposive, communication behavior that is intention based.

ACTIVE PURPOSIVE BEHAVIOR

By using the natural setting, the child's language can be used to obtain personally desired objects, to receive someone's action or help, to acquire the attention or presence of another person, and most important to help involve the child in the context for environmental learning. Parents, teachers, and uninformed bystanders (such as dentists) have reported an increase in the child's curiosity and general awareness of the environment when the child realized that utterances could change the hearer in some observable manner.

A preschool teacher of language impaired children incorporated these ideas into her classroom because she was tired of her children being passive to an adult environment. She video-recorded one of the first sessions in which she removed the chairs from the room. These typically nontalkative children explored, asked questions, and manipulated the context in all sorts of ways because they had a purpose for using their language to find their chairs. The children did find the chairs after much discussion and asking. The teacher had no intention of letting any of the children begin work without the chairs, and the only way they could get the chairs was through the performance of speech acts.

Expectations are part of the purpose for using language. If a speaker expects to receive the desired effects, then there's a purpose for speaking. If a speaker doesn't expect the desired effects, then there's no purpose. Once participating as a speaker, the child can begin the active process of learning from using language. The child's language structures further acquisition of higher level skills and lead to more language development. The child's undesired behaviors (although possibly showing an initial increase) are eventually replaced by a more social and therefore more desirable behavior, language.

The following examples highlight the importance of communication through an active linguistic process. If a child is to become part of the regular classroom, there are certain skills that are necessary in a busy setting. For example, the child must obtain help from the teacher in a conventional manner—that is, by raising a hand. Hand raising in this context signals the hearer that the child has something to say and is ready to speak. One special education child could do the academic skills required in regular classes but could not obtain the teacher's help, so the child would take off her clothes or be verbally abusive or both. By teaching the child the essential element (raising the hand) as part of the speech act, the child learned to stay in the classroom.

Many children are punished for "acting out" behavior such as being verbally abusive or physically manipulative or a class clown. But many of these behaviors could be rechanneled into direct linguistic skills for accomplishing the same effects: attention, assistance, objects, actions, and so forth. Children who are echolalic often respond quickly to this type of approach because anything that is said generates an observable consequence. The echolalia diminishes as the performance of speech acts increases. A child who is talkative—whether it's echolalic, tangential, off-topic, or abusive—remains a passive being, unless the child is an effective manipulator by linguistic means.

SUPPLEMENTAL MODES

There has been some previous mention of supplemental or alternate modes. (For this discussion, the term supplemental will be used since the additional mode is used for teaching and for learning.) Until the child is put in the position of being the speaker and the hearer, the child is not acquiring language that will improve learning. There may be, and probably is, some passive learning that continues to occur, but the advanced conceptual skills need organization of thought, whether through a vocal or nonvocal mode. If a child is beyond 24 months in age and is not using linguistic skills, one or two-term semantic relations, then the child's development is being affected. Whether this effect is permanent or temporary, there are changes occurring in the child's learning environment. Therefore, some effort should be made to set the contexts so that the child has a purpose or need for using language. This should greatly enhance the child's learning of the language system.

By the time the child is three years old or there is a diagnosed problem which is known to affect the child's language development (such as Down's Syndrome), the child should be given the opportunity to express needs or perform nonvocal acts intended to change adults and children in some desired manner. Although the mode (for example, sign language) may be nonvocal, the concepts developing the semantic relations and functions may still be expressed in nonvocal acts that change the context. But the vocal portion need not be omitted, so the visual method is a supplement to the auditory channel. For the children that have been given supplemental modes in this approach, the desire to communicate mushrooms and so does the desire to use vocal linguistic skills.

The use of any language skills is paramount to the child's learning and academic growth. Therefore, there cannot be too great an emphasis on providing a supplemental mode. It is never too late to try to begin the visual channel, nor is it ever too early. The method is the same as for the auditory channel. The same suggestions and procedures are used, with the child receiving the same input, but combined in a visual and auditory channel. The child's needs must still be expressed, and the child must have those needs met if the child is to have a purpose for communicating.

GOALS AND OBJECTIVES

The primary goal for the children enrolled in this remediation program is to be able to perform a variety of speech acts in a variety of contexts. Although data taking procedures provide the best assessment of whether the goal has been accomplished, pre- and post-testing with the BISAP is feasible.

The objectives for this procedure are divided into the specific speech acts (that is, the child's ability to perform requests for objects, for example) and into levels of spontaneity. A true performance of a speech act, by definition, implies initiation. But with the cues and imitation models, the child may be able to request with imitation (one objective) but not with just direct cues. So another objective would be moving from imitation to direct cues to spontaneous production.

The criteria for moving on to the next level can be measured by a percentage of consistency or frequency of speech acts in a given amount of time with a given number of opportunities. For example, in ten opportunities a child produced three speech acts by imitation for a 30 percent consistency by imitation, with a zero baseline for direct cues (assumed that the process of direct cues are provided in all ten opportunities), and a zero baseline for spontaneous performances. A percentage of consistency may be obtained for any speech act at any level of complexity.

Data Accountability

The recording of data is an important and inevitable part of the therapy process. An observer viewing the children in this setting may believe that the setting is nonstructured and is not effective or as accountable as a training context. On the contrary, any therapy setting or learning environment must have certain intrinsic components:

1. The context must have *internal control or structure*. The clinician or educator must know what is being taught, how it is being taught, when it has been taught, what to teach next, and what the final product is to be. For example: for this setting speech act performance is being taught; the opportunities, models, and cues are part of the process to teach speech act performance; when the child is capable of producing the desired types of speech acts, then the goal has been met through the objectives; the levels

of difficulty depend on the amount of cueing and modeling needed for the various types of speech acts in varying contexts; and the final product is a child who is an effective speaker—that is, someone who can convey an intended message to a hearer in order to alter the hearer's attitudes, beliefs, and behaviors.

2. The context must have *external control or structure*. The materials must be the best materials for facilitating the desired behavior, the setting must contain the best variables for facilitating the behavior, the teacher must use the techniques with maximum efficiency to obtain the maximum number of performances from the child, and the data must reflect an accurate picture of the therapy setting.

3. The data taking must be *accountable* to the child and to the adult. The data must reflect the child as that child truly is on most occasions and not as the child is during an isolated sample. The data must reflect what effect the adult has on the child's learning in order to demonstrate the value of the adult's presence. Chapter 9 discusses accountability as a general function of educational intervention for language disorders. Table 8-1 illustrates one method of data taking for this approach.

Table 8-1 Data Taking Procedures for Speech Acts

Speech Acts	
Request Action	√ P √ P √ P √ P
Request Object	√ P √ P √ P √ F √ F √ P √ P √ F √ F √ P
Request Information	√ P √ P √ P P P
Assertion	√ P P P (3 cues) √ P P P I (3 cues, finally imitation)
Statement of Information	
Rule Ordering	
Denial	
Calling	

Child:	Carl	Key:	√ speech act
Activity:	Academic work		√ P indirect cue
Time:	9:00-9:30		√ F imitation
Date:	11/12/80		o opportunity—cues and imitation do not help

This table illustrates that the data are organized by speech act, number, and type of preceding event or antecedent. This data should provide the clinician with enough information to determine the level of difficulty and what the next step in the intervention should be. For most young children, the speech acts that occur with the highest frequency are the requests, assertions, and rule orderings. The data are obtained for a selected period of time. After the data have been taken for that period, it may be decided that the data are not representative. In that case it is probably most accurate to take the average for several samplings.

The percentages of the number of speech acts that are performed or attempted should increase. If the child could consistently and appropriately manipulate the environment through speech acts, then there would be no need for this intervention. If the child can't do this, then therapy should improve the child's performance.

SUMMARY

A child who is not capable of performing speech acts as determined by behavioral observations, anecdotal records, and the Behavioral Inventory of Speech Act Performances should be put into therapy or educational (includes home) settings that provide the models and cues necessary to direct the child through the successful speech acts.

Questions

1. Why does facilitation of language usage improve other types of linguistic skills?
2. When should this type of program be implemented?
3. Why is a speech act an important feature of communication?
4. What units other than the speech act may be used for facilitating pragmatic language skills?
5. Why is pragmatics (the use of language for communication) considered a determining property in the acquisition of syntax, morphology, semantics, and phonology?

REFERENCES

Bates, E. Pragmatics and sociolinguistics in child language. In D. M. Morehead & A. E. Morehead (Eds.), *Normal and deficient child language*. Baltimore, Md.: University Park Press, 1976.

Brown, M. *Speech act types in three year old children*. Unpublished manuscript, Washington State University, 1979.

Bruner, J. S. The ontogenesis of speech acts. *Journal of Child Language*, 1974, *2*, 1-19.

Dore, J. The development of speech acts. (Doctoral dissertation, City University of New York, 1973). *Dissertation Abstracts International*, 1973, *34*. (University Microfilms No. 73-14, 374).

Hoag, L. *Application of speech act theory to language disordered children: The program*. Unpublished manuscript, University of Illinois, 1975.

Lucas, E. V. The feasibility of speech acts as a language approach for emotionally disturbed children. (Doctoral dissertation, University of Georgia, 1977). *Dissertation Abstracts International*, 1978, *38*, 3479B-3967B. (University Microfilms No. 77-30, 488).

Mundell, C., & Lucas, E. *A parent conducted pragmatic language program for Down's Syndrome children*. An unpublished manuscript, Washington State University, 1978.

CHAPTER OBJECTIVES

- explain the variables of internal accountability.

- explain the variables of external accountability.

- discuss the relationship of external to internal accountability.

- explain the significance of data taking as it relates to accountability and professional responsibility.

- explain the significance of content validity as it relates to assessment procedures and subsequent therapy for language disorders.

- explain the significance of progress for a child in language therapy and explain the accountability variables.

- explain the variables of progress related to individual variance, such as technique execution.

- provide a rationale for considering accountability as part of the remediation process.

- explain the variables that influence whether remediation programs have lasting effects or short-term or immediate effects.

- explain the importance of the initial assessment and how it relates to evaluating the child's progress in the remediation program.

Chapter 9

Accountability Procedures

*The validity of one's measure is not in the
represented numbers but in the
absolute value of its existence.*

The remediation procedures described in this book are only as effective as the assessment and only as efficient as the practitioners' abilities to implement them when appropriate.

There are a variety of procedures one can use to evaluate a child's progress, and to a lesser extent, a variety of methods available for critiquing the teacher's or clinician's effectiveness. Those data taking procedures used to represent the child's or adult's progress relate to the *external accountability*. *Internal accountability* refers to the therapist's understanding of the rationale of the remediation program as it relates to current research. Without both kinds of accountability, the child may be making immediate gains that do not represent an overall improvement in the child's communicative competence, the ultimate goal of the therapy.

INTERNAL ACCOUNTABILITY

Internal accountability can be arbitrarily divided into the following issues: (1) theoretical basis; (2) assessment basis; and (3) chosen approach. Each of these issues should address critical evaluation questions to the satisfaction of those individuals involved with the child. Through this kind of evaluation, the educator or clinician can be sure that the goals and objectives of the remediation program have been mastered in the most effective and efficient manner.

223

Theoretical Basis

Attitudes and beliefs about the way language is acquired will influence the methods or techniques chosen for remediation with a specific child. For example, if a person believes that language consists of a series of processes that may be taught, then the child's language therapy would probably consist of teaching "auditory and/or visual processing skills."

There are some problems that result from this logical matching of theoretical basis to program development.

The area of language meaning and usage cannot be matched to the theoretical operations that imply process development and/or unit building. Language skills represent a series of processes that function simultaneously and not independently. These processes are not hierarchical in the nature of being learned, since they are present in very young children; but the processes are hierarchical in complexity when combined. Therefore, work on separate processes or separate units will not build into ultimate adult communicative competence. (Children have a basic or rudimentary communicative competence at a very early age.) It is the expression or tools for expression that gain flexibility and power during the first year of language development.

If it is important that the child *talk better* and be *better understood,* then a therapy program based on the pieces that are believed to be involved with language development may never help the child become communicatively competent. Those processes and tasks that represent the processing skills may influence a child's ability to perform similar academic tasks. However, the processes function simultaneously in language and only then is the complexity issue significant to language therapy. For this book, the theoretical premise is that a very young child is capable of communicating an intent through linguistic skills that expand in complexity. Therefore, remediation is centered around the teaching of ways to express intentions through expansion of linguistic skills. The speech act is used to convey (through linguistic and nonlinguistic behavior) an intent to a hearer whose attitudes, beliefs, and/or behaviors may be altered.

Similar to the problem posed by teaching processes is the problem of teaching any single unit. The unit analysis, smaller than a speech act, provides an insight into the complexity of the language, but the surface structures taken at face value undermine the semantic complexity and the child's cognitive dimension. The acquisition of structures will not result in linguistic communication for a purpose unless the prerequisites for the surface representation have been adequately developed.

The following questions should be asked by any clinician or educator prior to and/or during intervention to determine whether or not the theoretical basis is suitable for the therapy:

1. What are the tenets of the theoretical base being used?
2. Do these tenets match the expected outcome or long-range goals?
3. If there is no theoretical base, what is the rationale?
4. How do the tenets of the theoretical base meet the current knowledge of normal development?

If these questions are not satisfactorily answered, a reevaluation of the process is in order. For the therapy suggestions in this book, the answers are as follows:

1. The principles of the theoretical basis are the same as the principles for the theoretical speech act; that is, linguistic behavior is semantically rule governed as an active communicative process that has purpose and intent.
2. The expected outcome of the process is a child who can use a variety of speech acts by conventional means to convey intent.
3. The rationale for the theoretical framework is that the child's semantic basis must be firm for establishing the complex means of expressing the child's ideas.
4. The speech act principles and components match with the recent research in semantic development and the function or purpose of language acquisition (psycholinguistics and sociolinguistics).

Assessment

Clinicians and assessment teams often select instruments that are inexpensive, convenient to use, available, and popular without considering the theoretical basis or content validity of the instrument. The theoretical basis of the test is usually founded on the assumption that the items should represent a correlational value to what is being measured. The content validity asks the question, "Does the test measure what it is suppose to measure?" Unfortunately, most maturational items that depend on learning will correlate with the first years of chronological development (Bledsoe, 1972). Therefore, it's easy to have test items that can't adequately answer the content validity question. Language tests should assess components of language as defined. This book accepts the definition that language is a rule-based system of conventional symbols or language—more specifically, that language is syntax, morphology, semantics, phonology, and the use of these (that is, pragmatics).

By definition, language test items that have a high content validity should assess phonology, semantics, morphology, and syntax, as well as the use of these. Therefore, a test that includes an item for drawing or copying would not be a test that assesses only language but a test that assesses other skills that probably correlate with the maturational component of language—that is, they both proceed through developmental refinements.

The following questions should be asked to determine the content validity of assessment tools:

1. What skills do the individual items of the test assess?
2. How many of these items are for language?
3. How many of these items are for motor skills, gross and fine?
4. How many items test academic or readiness skills?
5. How many items test social skills?
6. How many items test self-help skills?
7. Does your instrument assess language or language *and* other skills?
8. Does the composite or final score reflect language skills only, or does it reflect developmental skills highly correlated with language?

For further discussion of content validity and various assessment variables of language, the reader is referred to Muma's (1973) discussion. For this book, the basic assumption of the qualitative language sample analysis and the criterion-referenced measures is that the problematic or deviant aspects of a child's language are directly analyzed for placement in remediation programs. Therefore, the content validity of these measures is directly correlated with the definition of language.

The assessment of language for children with language disorders is sensitive to the verbal component of most tests, that is to the directions and materials. The child with a moderate to severe language delay and/or disorder will not perceive the materials nor understand the directions as do other children the same age. Therefore, for the language disordered child the test measures aspects of ability other than language. For example, a receptive picture vocabulary test requires pointing to a picture but the stimulus is verbal, which may result in lower than representative scores. Similarly, verbal intelligence tests or tests that have complex verbal directions will affect the language disordered child's ability to perform on the test. The results of these measures must be carefully considered and periodically reevaluated, particularly during the preschool years of development.

The development of adaptive scales and ongoing evaluations have replaced the notion of a one-time diagnostic evaluation. Litigation requiring periodic evaluations of children's abilities has also encouraged the intermediate evaluation process. Again, if the diagnostician does not select content valid measurement tools, the periodic evaluation won't provide the best picture of what the child is capable or is not capable of doing. Effectiveness of the tools, regardless of the extent and time for assessment, is dependent on the usefulness of the chosen tool.

When the assessment is complete, the clinician or educator should have enough information to begin therapy. If the clinician must do additional assessment after the diagnostic evaluation, then there is a discrepancy between the chosen assessment tools and the clinician's approach. General assessment questions might include the following:

1. Does the assessment tool examine the areas of responsibility?
2. Is the assessment coverage adequate for determining therapeutic placement and program development?
3. Does the assessment provide sufficient information about the child as compared with other children?
4. Does the assessment provide information about this child's particular skills?

Chosen Approach

The chosen remediation approach is often based on the theoretical basis that underlies the assessment tool. This means that the clinician is apt to work on only those weaknesses described by a particular test. If other areas of ability are not assessed, then it is unlikely that the clinician will consider these other areas for remediation.

Sometimes tests that are prerequisites to entrance into a particular program for language remediation are used as the major assessment tool. The pretest and program placement assumption ignores any other possibilities, unless the program considers all aspects of language development.

There are some problems inherent in selecting a remediation approach based on test results developed from a particular theoretical perspective. Unless the testing generates feedback on all possible aspects of language, the child may not receive therapy for the language problem that is most significant. If the clinician or evaluation team uses tests that provide extra information about the child (in addition to the language measurements), the extra information is great. But if the test emphasizes extraneous measures and not language, then it will be difficult to develop a therapy program. For example, if the clinician knows that a child has difficulty with central auditory processing, it should suggest that therapy for language development should capitalize on visual strengths while compensating or improving the weak auditory skills. However, strengthening the auditory component may never improve the way the child uses linguistic skills to express ideas. Therefore, the remediation approach should be chosen on the basis of the child's needs as determined by content valid tests consistent with the theoretical basis for choosing the assessment.

The approach, although based on a theoretical position, should be adapted to the child's individual needs. For example, research literature from normal developmental studies suggests that the majority of children produce present progressive verb forms (*verb* + *ing*) prior to the future verb construction (*be form* + *verb*). This does not mean that every child will follow this pattern, nor should a child be placed on one type of task learning until he or she can do the prearranged tasks. Many language disordered children skip skill levels, a behavior consistent with the idea that a disorder is often nonsequential and/or nonsystematic. Many of these language disordered children can perform skills at a higher level than expected. For example, there are nonverbal—or more appropriately nonvocal—children who have acquired a sight vocabulary and limited reading skills even though they use little if any intelligible or purposive speech. One cannot ignore these higher level skills. The ultimate goal of the language therapy approach is communicative competence. The mode of communication should be chosen for the child's needs, not for the convenience of the clinician or educator.

One reason to check internal accountability is to assure those individuals involved with a child's educational programming that their child is being fully served. Daily data may show some progress on individual items, but the items must be additive so that there's a positive overall affect on the child's communicative abilities. For example, learning to repeat digits or putting squares in square holes are not skills that can develop in complexity so as to make a child a competent speaker. However, these tasks and skills may have a cumulative effect and improve other areas of development.

EXTERNAL ACCOUNTABILITY

External accountability may be arbitrarily divided into the following topics: (1) measurement of real change; (2) daily versus long-term effects; and (3) the efficacy of remediation.

Measurement of real changes refers to taking data on behaviors or skills that are making a difference in the child's daily functioning. If there is supposed to be a change in the child's ability to communicate, then data should be taken on those behaviors that will show these effects. Data may be recorded on an hourly, daily, weekly, or monthly basis for specific task abilities. Unfortunately, sometimes the children *don't get better*, but daily or short-term data are always showing progress. The discrepancy between long- and short-term effects depends on the following variables: the child, whether the intervention is actually changing significant behaviors, and/or if skills or tasks are being learned. If the child is learning skills, then there should be changes in other areas; if the child is only learning tasks, then the child will do well on the tasks but there won't be any long-term positive effect.

The final point regarding external accountability deals with the efficacy of remediation. Most remediation or habilitation programs do produce changes, but the time necessary to effect a change is also important. Changes produced during the language acquisition years capitalize on the child's maturation.

Evaluation Procedures

If the language intervention procedures are not making a difference, then there must be some reevaluation. There are several variables that play a part of the reevaluation procedure: (1) initial assessment of the child; (2) theoretical bases of the chosen approaches; (3) execution of the techniques; (4) evaluation of the effectiveness of the remediation program; and (5) changes in the child's own external and internal status.

For semantic and pragmatic language disorders, there are some specific points regarding the reevaluation. The therapy is only as effective as the clinician's initial assessment. This assessment—whether based on the language sample or on criterion referenced measures coupled with behavioral observations and standardized tests—assumes that the clinician fully understands normal language development or has had enough experience with native language learners to have an internal model for comparison. The more knowledge the clinician has about normal language skills and processes, the more likely it is that he or she will recognize specific problems, be able to pinpoint areas of remediation, and be able to plan the remediation program.

The theoretical basis for the semantic and pragmatic remediation procedures is tentative; more research in sociolinguistics and psycholinguistics is desperately needed, as well as a need to study what happens when the process isn't normal. The state of the art is commensurate with the research; as research is completed the issues will change and so will the theoretical bases and the remediation programs.

Even though numerous variables affect the overall progress and success of remediation or intervention, there is one basic principle: *The child should show genuine change toward the goal of communicative competence. If the child does not evidence this positive change, then the approach and the implementation should be reevaluated.*

Questions

1. Why do children often show immediate but not long-term changes from remediation programs?
2. Why do language programs vary in their philosophy of remediation?
3. What types of research questions need to be answered regarding the differences between normal and aberrant language acquisition?

4. Why haven't more studies that compare two or more remediation approaches been available?
5. Why are clinicians ultimately responsible for a child's language program?

REFERENCES

Bledsoe, J. C. *Essentials of educational research* (2nd ed.). Atlanta, Ga.: Optima House, 1972.

Muma, J. R. Language assessment: Some underlying assumptions. *ASHA*, 1973, *15* (7), 331-338.

Development of the Behavioral Inventory of Speech Act Performances

The purpose of the Behavioral Inventory of Speech Act Performances (BI-SAP) was to determine those linguistic and paralinguistic behaviors that normal children between the ages of 3 and 5 are able to demonstrate but that severely emotionally disturbed children fail to show under the same conditions.

The conditions were chosen specifically for the Rutland Center in order to maintain maximum participation by the emotionally disturbed children. Prior to the testing at Rutland, the Behavioral Inventory of Speech Act Performances was administered to 24 normal preschool children between the ages of 3-0 and 5-2 who were enrolled in the First Presbyterian Church Preschool, Athens, Georgia. Descriptive data and reliability measures were obtained from these administrations.

The descriptive data for the Behavioral Inventory of Speech Act performances has been tabled below:

$$N = 24 \qquad \sigma_T = .9324 \qquad \sigma_T^2 = .8696$$
$$\text{Range} = 48 = 51 \qquad \bar{X} = 50$$
$$\sigma_e^2 = .0262 \qquad \sigma_e = .1619$$

When a criterion referenced test is developed, the assumption is that there should be no variation among the true scores of the normal children. "These

---

Source: Lucas, E.V. The feasibility of speech acts as a language approach for emotionally disturbed children. (Doctoral dissertation, University of Georgia, 1977). *Dissertation Abstracts International,* 1978.

measures are intended not to discriminate among persons but to discriminate each person's score from a fixed-criterion score'' (Stanley, 1971, p. 435). For the purpose of developing the test, 51, the maximum score, was chosen as the criterion or expected score. Stanley (1971) provides a special formula developed by Livingston (1970) in which variance, covariance, and correlation in terms of the deviation of scores from the criterion (rather than from the mean) is used. The formula for the criterion referenced reliability coefficient developed by Livingston (1970) is

$$\rho_C^2(T_x, X) = \frac{\sigma_T^2 + (\mu_x - C_x)^2}{\sigma_x^2 + (\mu_x - C_x)^2}$$

μ_x is the mean score, and C is the criterion score. σ_T^2 is the variance of test scores. σ_x^2 is equal to $\sigma_T^2 + \sigma_e^2$. σ_e^2 is the variance of errors of measurement.

The obtained criterion referenced reliability was .986 where the mean is 50 and the criterion was 51. In this case, the reliability coefficient shows a strong interrelationship between the expected or criterion score and the obtained scores. In other words, the amount of group differences was quite small. Most of the children were able to perform most of the tasks.

The high reliability coefficient also indicates that the children did consistently well on the items. Out of the 51 items, only 6 different items were missed. The proportion of children who passed these six items are as follows: Item 4 was .96; item 16 was .96; item 23 was .96; item 26 was .75; item 27 was .92; and item 34 was .96. The errors were not age related since the three year olds passed 99 percent of all items; the four year olds passed 99 percent of all items; and the five year olds passed only 84 percent of all items. The only item that less than 90 percent passed was item 26 which requires the sequencing of three propositions for ''reporting.'' This item may reflect other factors outside of the test domain of speech acts, i.e., they are speech events. Glaser and Nitko (1971) suggest that the main problem in developing a criterion referenced test is to make sure that the test tasks are clearly members of the ''relevant domain.'' The investigator believes that an attempt to ''report'' a message has a distinct illocutionary force for a hearer.

One illocutionary force indicator that illustrates a report (without using a performative, ''I report'') is the sequencing of more than one proposition. To say one thing about a referent usually will leave the hearer with the effect from an assertion, whereas the summing of events provides a difficult effect. However, a linguistic requirement of three sequenced propositions probably contaminates the effect the speaker wants to convey with the syntactical ability to conjoin and the cognitive abilities of recall and temporal sequencing. Therefore, the ''relevant domain'' of speech act tasks may have been contaminated on item 26 by the different developmental levels of cognition and recall being represented in the normal children.

Even though the initial proportion of normal children passing item 26 was .75, item 26 was not deleted or changed for the emotionally disturbed children. None of the emotionally disturbed children passed item 26 on the pre-control and post-control measures. However, two of the children passed it on the post-intervention measures, indicating a possible growth in their ability to organize or sequence events as well as in their ability to use linguistic skills to "report."

Inter-Judge Reliability

Although the investigator administered all inventories to the 24 normal children as well as to the eight emotionally disturbed children used in the study, a percentage of other judges' reliability with the investigator was obtained. Three trained judges simultaneously rated and scored the performance of two normal preschool children. One hundred percent agreement was obtained, indicating a high inter-judge reliability.

REFERENCES

Livingston, S.A. The reliability of criterion-referenced measures. Center for Social Organization of Schools. *Technical Report,* The Johns Hopkins University, July 1970, No. 73.

Stanley, J.C. Reliability. In R.L. Thorndike (Ed.), *Educational Measurement* (2nd ed.). New York: American Council on Education, 1971.

Scoring Instructions of Essential Elements: Behavioral Inventory of Speech Act Performances

The Behavioral Inventory of Speech Act Performances (BISAP) is a performance test. Each speech act is performed in a situation or context requiring specific linguistic and paralinguistic elements for completion of an act. All tasks for eliciting the act are the same for all children and are presented in a structured setting with conversational dialogue. Each of the expected acts are divided into five or six elements considered most important or essential to the successful completion of the act. Each element present in the child's performance is to be checked under the "yes column" if it is present and under the "no column" if it is not present. All checks under the "yes column" are scored as one, and all checks under the "no column" are scored as 0. Therefore, the child's test score is equal to the total number of essential elements observed to be present in the child's performance. The maximum possible score on the test is 51.

The acts are arranged on the score sheet according to the presentation of the tasks. To score each task, place the test item sheet to the left of the score sheet. Below each task described on the item sheet is a number (e.g., 1.) corresponding to the act on the score sheet (e.g., 1. corresponds to requests). As soon as the examiner gives the verbal instruction to the child, the scorer should begin to judge whether or not the child uses the specific elements to complete the task. Each child has one minute to complete the task once the examiner has given the

Source: Lucas, E.V. The feasibility of speech acts as a language approach for emotionally disturbed children. (Doctoral dissertation, University of Georgia, 1977). *Dissertation Abstracts International,* 1978.

child the directions for the task. During this minute, the examiner may reword or restate the directions. Since the purpose of the tasks is to provide a context to determine if the child can perform specific acts, the degree or type of linguistic cues given by the examiner should vary with the different acts. For example, the presence of the picture, plus "tell me about your picture," may be enough context for eliciting an assertion. However, other acts such as "experiencing" require that the examiner offer more verbal cues to set the context for the child to give a "feeling" type of utterance.

Children should not be judged on their use of grammatical utterances (subject-verb agreement; use of articles; use of specific morphological markers such as *ed* to indicate past tense; use of prepositional phrases; confusions of pronouns, etc.). Children should be judged on their effectiveness in completing the tasks. In other words, the scorer is interested in how well the children communicated the meaning of their utterances during each task in terms of specific linguistic and paralinguistic elements described on the score sheet.

Score Sheet

Behavioral Inventory of Speech Act Performances

	Yes	No

1. Requests for objects (materials)
   a. S's body orientation is toward the H in order to ready H for the utterance.   1a
   b. Eye contact or name is used to signal H.   1b
   c. Appropriate linguistic markers indicating either   1c
      —an interrogative form, or
      —an imperative form.
   d. An utterance which specifies what the adult is to do.   1d
   e. Appropriate loudness for the listener to respond.   1e
2. Requests for action (draw)
   a. S's body orientation is toward H in order to ready H for the utterance.   2a
   b. Eye contact or name is used to signal H.   2b
   c. Appropriate linguistic markers indicating either   2c
      —an interrogative form, or
      —an imperative form.
   d. An utterance which specifies what the adult is to do.   2d
   e. Appropriate loudness for the listener to respond.   2e
3. Assertion (about picture)
   a. A falling contour representative of a declarative form.   3a
   b. A form of __ is X, which does not follow by direct imitation.   3b
   c. The utterance is given with appropriate loudness.   3c
   d. Eye contact is given to signal the H, or observation is given to signal H.   3d
   e. Body orientation between S and H within a front plane position.   3e
4. Denial (to draw complicated picture)
   a. The previous action (or p of the H) is implied through gesture or is linguistically specified.   4a
   b. Use of emphatic stress or loudness for H to respond.   4b

c. The utterance is negatively marked.   4c
d. Eye contact is used to signal H.   4d
e. Orientation is toward the H or toward the action or materials being denied.   4e

5. Statements of information (what child did first)
   a. Falling contour representative of a declarative form.   5a
   b. Appropriate loudness for the H to respond.   5b
   c. Content is factual for the H.   5c
   d. Eye contact signals the H, or observation signals the H.   5d
   e. Orientation of the body is toward H.   5e

6. Requests for information (making picture)
   a. The utterance is marked with a rising contour.   6a
   b. The utterance utilizes a specific lexical item indicating a constituent question, or an interrogative reversal indicating the answer to a yes/no question.   6b
   c. Appropriate loudness is used for the listener to respond.   6c
   d. Eye contact signals H, or observation signals H.   6d
   e. Body orientation is either toward the materials or toward H.   6e

7. Calling or summons
   a. The H is specified by name or signaled by some other linguistic marker of notification.   7a
   b. Orientation is facing H.   7b
   c. Eye contact or observation is made during or as a part of the utterance.   7c
   d. The utterance specifies how the H is to perform or respond.   7d
   e. The loudness is adequate for H to respond.   7e

8. Rule order (What the teacher is to do)
   a. The utterance is given with a falling contour of an imperative form.   8a
   b. The utterance is given with adequate loudness for H to respond.   8b
   c. Body orientation is toward H.   8c
   d. Eye contact signals H, or observation signals H.   8d
   e. The utterance specifies what H is to do.   8e

Experiences and reports have been deleted. Total is 40.

Art Context for the Behavioral Inventory of Speech Act Performances

Context: The context for the inventory includes a familiar teacher and the investigator working with each child on an individual basis in the Rutland Center art room. Each child is told that he or she will be leaving the regular classroom three times in one term to do these tasks. All children are praised for their participation in these art tasks. No child is allowed to experience failure, since the tasks are solved by the hearer in one minute or less depending on the child's needs.

Task 1: Requests for objects
  The child is told to choose the materials from the teacher that he or she wants to use for drawing a picture. The teacher is turned away from the child so that the child does not think the teacher knows what he or she wants.
Task 2: Requests for action
  Once the child has attempted to receive his or her materials from the teacher, or one minute has elapsed, a suggestion is made to the child to get the teacher to draw a picture.
Task 3: Assertion
  Either upon request to tell something about the previously drawn picture or after the child draws a picture, the investigator asks the child to tell something about the picture.

Source: Lucas, E. V. The feasibility of speech acts as a language approach for emotionally disturbed children. (Doctoral dissertation, University of Georgia, 1977). *Dissertation Abstracts International, 1978.*

Task 4: Denial

After the assertion of one minute, the teacher asks the child to draw a very difficult picture the child does not know how to draw or does not think he or she knows how to draw (e.g., draw a stegosaurus).

Task 5: Statements of information

Once the child has attempted to deny the requests, or one minute has passed, the teacher asks the child what he or she did first when coming into the art room.

Task 6: Reporting (speech event)

Once the child has given a statement of information, then he or she is verbally cued to tell more about his or her day.

Task 7: Requests for information

Once the child has attempted to report, or enough time has passed to indicate an attempt, the child is shown a picture covered with a solid color paint and a picture showing an etching. The child is asked to make an etching for the teacher. In order to know how to make the etching, the child must request more information since he or she is given no tool or cues as to how the picture was made.

For the second testing occasion, a paper cut-out design is used. For the third testing occasion, an erasable slate is used.

Task 8: Experiencing (speech event)

After the child is shown how to complete the previous task, either by requests cr by the teacher, the teacher asks the child how he or she feels and if he or she wishes to continue the tasks.

Task 9: Calling

If the child wishes to continue with the previous tasks, the child may finish it. If he or she does not wish to continue, he or she is allowed to choose a new art task. The investigator then reminds the teacher that the teacher has some work to do. The teacher then explains to the child that the teacher is going outside to the waiting or observation room (whichever is appropriate for this child) and that the child is to come get the teacher when he or she is finished and say that it is time to go back to the classroom. After the child finishes the immediate art task, the investigator tells the child that they are finished. The child is reminded to go get the teacher and tell the teacher that it is time to go back to the classroom.

Task 10: Rule order

The child goes out and signals the teacher in some way (calling). Then the teacher waits momentarily to see if the child wants to go back to the classroom. If the child does not give the rule, the teacher asks the child if he or she is ready to go back to the room.

Glossary

Anomia—inability to recall (for use) the sign or specific lexical tag of a referent.

Auditory Misperception—inability to relate the phonetic representation and thus to correctly produce the attached symbolic sign; e.g., consistent production of bressed for dressed.

Boundaries—conventional set of phrasing markers such as terminal pause and stress indicators.

Communicative Competence—the speaker's ability to effectively communicate an intentional message so as to alter the hearer's attitudes, beliefs, and/or behaviors. Therefore, a very young child could be communicatively competent with a minimal development of linguistic skills.

Concept—organization of percepts into referential meaning.

Connotative Meaning—implied meaning separate from the word's designated meaning.

Constituent—a referent omitted in the linguistic pattern but understood through contextual features and shared past experiences. "What" is the referent omitted in the constituent question, "What is that?"

Constitutive Rules—hypothetical semantic rules regulating the speech act.

Contentives—content bearing words (usually represented by nouns, verbs, and adjectives) that have referential meaning.

Contour—the overall intonation pattern of an utterance that indicates a rising or falling terminal marker.

241

Cues—teaching devices used to focus an individual's attention on a task (for example, visual, tactile, and auditory cues).

Deixis—social interchange facilitating language acquisition through sharing the reciprocal roles of speaker and hearer.

Denotative Meaning—the specific meanings related to an individual word.

Echolalia—vocal repetition of previously heard utterances, phrases, and sentences.

Facilitation—habilitative methods used to assist the acquisition of the sequential and systematic pattern of language.

Fillers—words or syllables uttered in place of a referent.

Function—the intended effect of the message on the hearer.

Functors—the lexical terms used to expand referential meaning (for example, terms such as "the," "a," or "on").

Illocutionary Act—uttering sounds or symbols said to have meaning in the speaker's intentions and in a subsequent effect on the hearer.

Illocutionary Force Indicators—those devices that determine how the hearer takes the proposition. In English these devices include word order, stress, intonation contour, the mood of the verb, performative verbs, and punctuation.

Indefinite Terms or Modifiers—words that receive their referential meaning from only the environmental or linguistic context (for example, "it," "they," or "one").

Intervention—prescriptive teaching aimed at altering the present course of learning language.

Labeling—the attachment of signs and/or symbols to referents for the purpose of naming. (Labeling usually is not evident in adult language.)

Language—a system of symbols agreed upon by two or more people and governed by the linguistic properties inherent in phonology, syntax, morphology, and semantics.

Language Age—a child's level of language development as compared to the expected development of a child of the same chronological age. For example, a chronological age of 4.0 should be the same as the language age, 4.0.

Language Delay—systematic and sequential delay in the acquisition of linguistic skills.

Language Disorder—a nonsystematic and nonsequential development of language and/or the presence of specific disorders.

Lexical Tags—the word or verbal symbols associated with the referent.

Lexicon—the vocabulary or morphemes of a language, or the specific repertoire of vocabulary for a specific individual.

Linguistic Competence—the native speaker's set of rules for generating and understanding conventional structures that are meaningfully appropriate.

Locutionary Act—uttering words plus the content of the message.

Mark (Marker, Marking)—the lexical tag or linguistic form of the morphemes.

Model—a speaker who produces utterances that exemplify forms to be imitated or improved upon by the speaker.

Modulations—morphemic changes by suffixes or inflectional morphemes used to specify or denote changes in meaning.

Morpheme—basic unit of meaning that generally is considered in free (referential meaning) and bound (specify or modulate referents) forms.

Morphology—study of the morpheme, a basic unit of meaning as it is derived and combined to change referential meanings, for example, the addition of -s for plural, and so forth.

Morphophonemic Rules—these rules combine the morphemes and phonemes into surface representation.

Neologisms—an individual's creation of an unconventional word or lexical tag.

Off Target Responding—the speaker's utterances lack the expected connection with conversational referents resulting in a production that does not meet existing propositional content expectations.

Paradigmatic Association—a word class association such as "red" associates to "yellow" or "apple" associates to "table."

Paralinguistic—vocal and nonverbal indices (such as breath pause or eye contact) that add meaning or clarification to an utterance.

Pause—breath markers meaningfully separating ideas or propositions sometimes exaggerated by the speaker to highlight a specific idea.

Performatives—prelinguistic motor acts that represent a communicative intent but more commonly the verbs that signify an active process (e.g., marry, swear, pledge, etc.).

Perlocutionary Act—the effects of specific acts on a hearer.

Personalness—a semantic feature related to the individual's self.

Phonological Disorder—a nonsystematic and nonsequential development of the conventional sound system.

Phonology—the study of the acquisition, comprehension, and production of conventional sound rules used to code the form or structure.

Pragmatics—the use of syntax, morphology, semantics, and phonology to convey an intended message to alter the attitudes, beliefs, or behaviors of a hearer.

Predication—occurs in the form of X is Y, where X is the idea of the utterance and Y is the comment or predication of the utterance. The predication or argument (universal term) expands on the specific term of the utterance.

Primitive Speech Acts—term coined by Dore (1974) to indicate a child's attempt to produce a speech act.

Propositional Act—the meaning or content of the utterance consisting of referring and/or predicating. The propositional act occurs with the illocutionary act.

Prosody—paralinguistic vocal features particularly of tonal quality but not limited.

Redirection—a verbal or nonverbal method designated to keep a child on task.

Referent—an object, action, or event that may be specified and thus denoted or tagged in meaning.

Referential Meaning—explicit meaning expressed by lexicon developed through shared experiences.

Referring—specifying or marking an object, action, or event through linguistic terms.

Semantic Features—characteristics contributing to the concept; these may be grouped into two major types of attributes: perceptual or functional.

Semantic Functions—the purpose of an utterance or the speaker's intention.

Semantic Relations—implied meaning by association or interaction of meaningful notions such as agents, actions, and objects as in relationships; e.g. agent + object.

Semantic Sequencing—the conventional ordering of propositions according to spatio-temporal concepts.

Semantic Word Errors—unconventional use of lexical tags.

Spatial—refers to orientation of the child in relationship to others and to environmental objects and events.

Speech Act—Searle (1969) hypothesized that the speech act is the basic unit of communication which includes "what the speaker means, what the sentence (or other linguistic elements) uttered means, what the speaker intends, what the hearer understands, and what the rules governing the linguistic elements are" (p. 21). Speech acts include making promises, statements, requests, assertions, etc.

Speech Event—a series of speech acts about a proposition uttered in a given context.

Syntactic Error—typically an error in word order. This book suggests that some syntactic errors (surface representation) are part of a semantic disorder.

Syntagmatic Association—the association follows a syntactic order. For example, "red" might be associated to any noun that might follow the adjective.

Syntax—the conventional ordering of the lexicon into grammatical structures.

Tangential Utterance—the topic of this utterance is an association to the immediate referents.

Temporal—refers to the sequence of events by time.

Topic Closure—the speaker usually determines the boundaries of the conversation so that the first topic may be finished before continuing on to the second, third, fourth, etc.

Utterance Act—actual production of sounds to represent ideas.

Verbal Perseveration—a verbal repetition of a self-produced and novel sentence, phrase, and/or word.

Index

Note: Page numbers in italics designate tables.

About the Author

ELLYN V. LUCAS received her doctorate from the University of Georgia in speech and language pathology. She has been a clinical supervisor at the University of Illinois and at the University of Georgia and has worked with a wide range of language delayed and language disordered children. As an assistant professor at Washington State University, she taught courses in language development, language disorders and methods, diagnostics, and psycholinguistics. Dr. Lucas has published and presented numerous articles and papers that emphasize her clinical work in the application of psycholinguistic and sociolinguistic literature. She has conducted and directed inservice and workshop programs focusing on language methods and procedures. Presently, Dr. Lucas is an assistant professor in speech pathology and audiology at Texas Tech University, Lubbock, Texas.